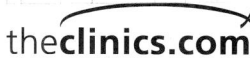

RHEUMATIC DISEASE CLINICS OF NORTH AMERICA

Early Rheumatoid Arthritis

GUEST EDITOR
Paul Emery, MA, MD, FRCP

November 2005 • Volume 31 • Number 4

SAUNDERS

An Imprint of Elsevier, Inc.
PHILADELPHIA   LONDON   TORONTO   MONTREAL   SYDNEY   TOKYO

W.B. SAUNDERS COMPANY
A Division of Elsevier Inc.

1600 John F. Kennedy Boulevard • Suite 1800 • Philadelphia, Pennsylvania 19103-2899

http://www.theclinics.com

RHEUMATIC DISEASE
CLINICS OF NORTH AMERICA   Volume 31, Number 4
November 2005   ISSN 0889-857X
Editor: Barton Dudlick   ISBN 1-4160-2767-X

The ideas and opinions expressed in *Rheumatic Disease Clinics of North America* do not necessarily reflect those of the Publisher. The Publisher does not assume any responsibility for any injury and/or damage to persons or property arising out of or related to any use of the material contained in this periodical. The reader is advised to check the appropriate medical literature and the product information currently provided by the manufacturer of each drug to be administered to verify the dosage, the method and duration of administration, or contraindications. It is the responsibility of the treating physician or other health care professional, relying on independent experience and knowledge of the patient, to determine drug dosages and the best treatment for the patient. Mention of any product in this issue should not be construed as endorsement by the contributors, editors, or the Publisher of the product or manufacturers' claims.

Rheumatic Disease Clinics of North America (ISSN 0889-857X) is published quarterly by Elsevier Inc. Corporate and editorial offices: 1600 John F. Kennedy Boulevard, Suite 1800, Philadelphia, PA 19103-2899. Accounting and circulation offices: 6277 Sea Harbor Drive, Orlando, FL 32887-4800. Periodicals postage paid at Orlando, FL 32862, and additional mailing offices. Subscription prices are USD 190 per year for US individuals, USD 305 per year for US institutions, USD 95 per year for US students and residents, USD 225 per year for Canadian individuals, USD 370 per year for Canadian institutions, USD 250 per year for international individuals, USD 370 per year for international institutions and USD 125 per year for Canadian and foreign students/residents. To receive student/resident rate, orders must be accompanied by name of affiliated institution, date of term, and the *signature* of program/residency coordinator on institution letterhead. Orders will be billed at individual rate until proof of status received. Foreign air speed delivery is included in all *Clinics* subscription prices. All prices are subject to change without notice. POSTMASTER: Send address changes to *Rheumatic Disease Clinics of North America*, W.B. Saunders Company, Periodicals Fulfillment, Orlando, FL 32887-4800. **Customer Service: 1-800-654-2452 (USA). From outside of the USA, call (+1) 407-345-4000. E-mail: hhspcs@harcourt.com.**

Reprints. For copies of 100 or more of articles in this publication, please contact the Commercial Reprints Department, Elsevier Inc., 360 Park Avenue South, New York, New York, 10010-1710; Tel.: (+1) 212-633-3813, Fax: (+1) 212-462-1935, and E-mail: reprints@elsevier.com.

Rheumatic Disease Clinics of North America is covered in *Index Medicus, Current Contents/ Clinical Medicine, Science Citation Index, ISI/BIOMED,* and *EMBASE/Excerpta Medica.*

Printed in the United States of America.

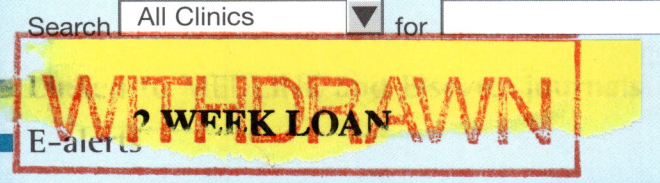
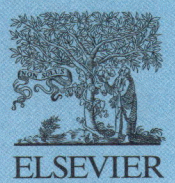

GUEST EDITOR

PAUL EMERY, MA, MD, FRCP, Arthritis Research Campaign Professor (Rheumatology); Head, Academic Unit of Musculoskeletal Disease, Rheumatology and Rehabilitation Research Unit, Chapel Allerton Hospital; and Clinical Director, Leeds Teaching Hospitals Trust, Leeds, United Kingdom

CONTRIBUTORS

ANNELIES BOONEN, MD, PhD, Rheumatologist, Division of Rheumatology, Department of Internal Medicine, University Hospital Maastricht and Care and Public Health Research Institute, University Maastricht, Maastricht, The Netherlands

FERDINAND C. BREEDVELD, MD, PhD, Head, Department of Rheumatology, Leiden University Medical Center; and Professor and Chairman, Department of Internal Medicine, Leiden, The Netherlands

ANDREW K. BROWN, MBChB, MRCP(UK), Lecturer, Academic Unit of Musculoskeletal Disease, Department of Rheumatology, Leeds General Infirmary, Leeds, United Kingdom

LORNA CAWKWELL, MRCP, Clinical Research Fellow (Rheumatology), Academic Unit of Musculoskeletal Disease, Chapel Allerton Hospital, Leeds, United Kingdom

PHILIP G. CONAGHAN, MBBS, PhD, FRACP, FRCP, Professor (Musculoskeletal Medicine), Academic Unit of Musculoskeletal Disease, Department of Rheumatology, Leeds General Infirmary, Leeds, United Kingdom

SALLY COX, BMBS, Research Fellow (Rheumatology), Academic Unit of Musculoskeletal Disease, Department of Rheumatology, Chapel Allerton Hospital, Leeds, United Kingdom

JOHN J. CUSH, MD, Chief, Department of Rheumatology and Clinical Immunology, Presbyterian Hospital of Dallas, Dallas, Texas

JESKA K. DE VRIES-BOUWSTRA, MD, Department of Rheumatology, VU University Medical Center, Amsterdam, The Netherlands

BEN A.C. DIJKMANS, MD, PhD, Professor and Head, Department of Rheumatology, VU University Medical Center, Amsterdam, The Netherlands

HANI S. EL-GABALAWY, MD, FRCPC, Professor, Department of Medicine, University of Manitoba and Arthritis Center, Winnipeg, Manitoba, Canada

PAUL EMERY, MA, MD, FRCP, Arthritis Research Campaign Professor (Rheumatology); Head, Academic Unit of Musculoskeletal Disease, Rheumatology and Rehabilitation Research Unit, Chapel Allerton Hospital; and Clinical Director, Leeds Teaching Hospitals Trust, Leeds, United Kingdom

MICHAEL J. GREEN, MRCP, Consultant Rheumatologist, Academic Unit of Musculoskeletal Disease, Chapel Allerton Hospital, Leeds; Harrogate and District NHS Foundation Trust, Harrogate; and York Hospital, York, United Kingdom

PEKKA HANNONEN, MD, PhD, Professor, Kuopio University; and Head, Department of Medicine, Jyväskylä Central Hospital, Jyväskylä, Finland

GLENN HAUGEBERG, MD, PhD, Consultant (Rheumatology), Department of Rheumatology, Sørlandet Hospital, Kristiansand; and Professor, Norwegian University of Science and Technology, Trondheim, Norway

CAROL A. HITCHON, MD, FRCPC, MSc, Assistant Professor, Department of Medicine, University of Manitoba and Arthritis Center, Winnipeg, Manitoba, Canada

DAVID KANE, PhD, MRCPI, Arthritis Research Campaign Clinical Senior Lecturer (Rheumatology), School of Clinical and Medical Sciences, University of Newcastle-upon-Tyne; and Musculoskeletal Department, Freeman Hospital, Newcastle-upon-Tyne, United Kingdom

HELEN I. KEEN, MBBS, FRACP, Research Fellow, Academic Unit of Musculoskeletal Disease, Department of Rheumatology, Leeds General Infirmary, Leeds, United Kingdom

HELENA MARZO-ORTEGA, MRCP, Specialist Registrar (Rheumatology), The Academic Unit of Musculoskeletal Disease, Chapel Allerton Hospital, Leeds, United Kingdom

TIMO MÖTTÖNEN, MD, PhD, Professor, Turku University; Department of Medicine, Turku University Central Hospital, Turku; and Division of Rheumatology, Paimio Hospital, Paimio, Finland

SANJAY PATHARE, MRCP(UK), Specialist Registrar (Rheumatology), Musculoskeletal Department, Freeman Hospital, Newcastle-upon-Tyne, United Kingdom

CHRISTINE A. PESCHKEN, MD, FRCPC, MSc, Assistant Professor, Department of Medicine, University of Manitoba and Arthritis Center, Winnipeg, Manitoba, Canada

MARK A. QUINN, MBChB, MRCP, Lecturer (Rheumatology), Academic Unit of Musculoskeletal Disease, Department of Rheumatology, Chapel Allerton Hospital, Leeds, United Kingdom

SAEED SHAIKH, MD, FRCPC, Department of Medicine, University of Manitoba and Arthritis Center, Winnipeg, Manitoba, Canada

TUULIKKI SOKKA, MD, PhD, Consultant Rheumatologist, Department of Rheumatology, Jyväskylä Central Hospital, Jyväskylä, Finland; and Research Assistant Professor, Department of Rheumatology, Vanderbilt University, Nashville, Tennessee

DÉSIRÉE VAN DER HEIJDE, MD, PhD, Professor, Division of Rheumatology, Department of Internal Medicine, University Hospital Maastricht and Care and Public Health Research Institute, University Maastricht, Maastricht, The Netherlands

RICHARD J. WAKEFIELD, BM, MRCP(UK), Senior Lecturer, Academic Unit of Musculoskeletal Disease, Department of Rheumatology, Leeds General Infirmary, Leeds, United Kingdom

ADAM YOUNG, MD, FRCP, Consultant Rheumatologist, City Hospital, St. Albans, Herts, United Kingdom

CONTENTS

Early Undifferentiated Arthritis

Carol A. Hitchon, Christine A. Peschken, Saeed Shaikh, and
Hani S. El-Gabalawy

Patients who cannot be classified as having a well-defined arthropathy typically are labeled as having undifferentiated arthritis. Some patients develop sufficient features to permit classification, whereas others remain undifferentiated, but with persistent joint inflammation, functional disability, and development of radiographic damage. Identifying the subset of patients destined to develop rheumatoid arthritis, spondyloarthropathy, or a more severe and persistent form of undifferentiated arthritis and choosing appropriate treatment strategies remain challenges for clinicians. Numerous investigative strategies are available with which to characterize undifferentiated arthritis and assess prognosis. This article discusses the characteristics of undifferentiated arthritis at presentation and the investigative strategies that can be used to predict prognosis and outcome early in the disease course. Therapeutic strategies also are explored.

Early Oligoarthritis

Helena Marzo-Ortega, Lorna Cawkwell, and Michael J. Green

Oligoarthritis is a common condition, with a variable outcome. It affects a predominantly young population and has a high morbidity when treated conventionally. The variability of outcome has limited the development of studies evaluating therapies such as disease-modifying antirheumatic drugs in recent onset disease. Oligoarthritis is an important disease that warrants much greater study.

Early Psoriatic Arthritis

David Kane and Sanjay Pathare

In the majority of patients with psoriatic arthritis (PsA), it is a chronic progressive disease, and only 12% of patients with early PsA will be in disease-modifying antirheumatic drug–free remission at 2 years. Radiologic damage occurs in the early stages of PsA; up to 47% of patients with PsA have radiologic erosions after 2 years. This article reviews the clinical features of early PsA, pathologic insights into PsA gleaned from studies of early PsA, and the current state of diagnostic imaging and therapeutics in early PsA.

Early Rheumatoid Arthritis

Adam Young

Longitudinal and observational studies have provided important information on the course of rheumatoid arthritis (RA), clinical outcomes, and prognostic markers. In terms of clinical effectiveness of drugs used in RA, the results of such projects can be used to complement those of randomized studies. If well designed and conducted, inception cohorts are the most robust types of observational studies, reflect the most complete spectrum of disease, and provide the most reliable prognostic markers for the management of this chronic condition.

Conventional X-Ray in Early Arthritis

Annelies Boonen and Désirée van der Heijde

This article reviews radiographic data from six cohorts of patients with early inflammatory arthritis. Radiographic scoring was not applied for diagnostic purposes but to detect damage as consequence synovitis with poor prognosis, in most studies rheumatoid arthritis. Class scoring methods were applied to detect and quantify damage. Of the patients, 8% to 15% had erosive disease at the first encounter with the rheumatologist, but baseline damage was low in early inflammatory arthritis. Yearly progression in damage score was assessed only in patients with high suspicion of rheumatoid arthritis at baseline or who had a final diagnosis of rheumatoid arthritis at follow-up and varied between 0.5% and 1.7% of the maximal damage of the scoring method per year. The large number of patients with zero values for erosions and lower progression rates will influence sample sizes in clinical trials in early inflammatory arthritis when including radiographic change as an outcome.

MRI and Musculoskeletal Ultrasonography as Diagnostic Tools in Early Arthritis

Helen I. Keen, Andrew K. Brown, Richard J. Wakefield, and Philip G. Conaghan

Rheumatoid arthritis (RA) is a chronic and progressive inflammatory disorder primarily affecting the synovium and is characterized by destruction of bone and cartilage. Early diagnosis and treatment of RA can improve disease outcomes substantially. Magnetic resonance imaging and musculoskeletal ultrasonography may facilitate early diagnosis and aid the targeting of intensive therapy. Magnetic resonance imaging and musculoskeletal ultrasonography also are able to monitor temporal changes in disease activity (ie, synovitis) and damage (ie, erosions). These imaging modalities are likely to be increasingly used in the management of early RA to ensure the best patient outcomes, although more work is required to determine their optimal roles.

Value of Dual-Energy X-Ray Absorptiometry as a Diagnostic and Assessment Tool in Early Rheumatoid Arthritis

Glenn Haugeberg and Paul Emery

New research has revealed common pathophysiologic and cellular mechanisms behind the development of osteoporosis and joint damage in rheumatoid arthritis (RA). Because osteoporosis is a direct consequence of the inflammatory disease process, bone mass measurements in principle could be an outcome marker of inflammation, of damage, and of response to therapeutic intervention. Several devices have been developed for quantitative bone mass assessment including dual-energy x-ray absorptiometry (DXA), which is considered the reference standard. This article, based on current data and understanding, discusses the use of DXA as a diagnostic and assessment tool especially in early RA.

Conventional Disease-Modifying Antirheumatic Drugs in Early Arthritis 729

Tuulikki Sokka, Pekka Hannonen, and Timo Möttönen

This article reviews the use of conventional disease-modifying antirheumatic drugs (DMARDs) in the treatment of early rheumatoid arthritis (RA). The Finnish early RA cohorts are used as examples of how early and active treatment strategies have improved over time with increasing variety of available DMARDs. Therapy goals of early RA include remission to prevent severe long-term outcomes of RA. Remission can be achieved in a third of patients with early RA using a combination of conventional DMARDs, including methotrexate, sulfasalazine, hydroxychloroquine, and prednisolone. Of patients with early RA, 20% to 30% do not improve enough with conventional treatments and should be identified at early phases to consider institution of biologic agents.

Biologics in Early Rheumatoid Arthritis 745

Jeska K. de Vries-Bouwstra, Ben A.C. Dijkmans, and Ferdinand C. Breedveld

Treatment of patients with rheumatoid arthritis (RA) with disease-modifying antirheumatic drugs is started immediately after diagnosis, resulting in more effective suppression of disease activity and substantial reduction of joint damage. The development of biologic agents has enabled remission as a realistic therapeutic goal in a greater proportion of patients. The tumor necrosis factor-α inhibitors, infliximab, etanercept, and adalimumab, have been studied in numerous randomized clinical trials. These agents can suppress disease activity directly, slow or stop progression of radiologic damage, and prevent further loss of quality of life. Patients treated with tumor necrosis factor-α inhibitors show few adverse events, which together with the high clinical effectiveness is favorable for treatment compliance. The exact role of these agents in the treatment of early-stage RA is unknown.

Potential for Altering Rheumatoid Arthritis Outcome 763

Mark A. Quinn and Paul Emery

The potential for disproportionately altering outcome in the early stages of rheumatoid arthritis (RA) was first hypothesized in the early 1990s. This window of opportunity hypothesis for therapeutic intervention in RA is based on the existence of a time frame within which there is a potential for a greater response to therapy, resulting in sustained benefits or, perhaps most important, a chance of cure. Given the persistent, progressive, damaging, inflammatory nature of RA, this approach to altering outcome in the early stages seems attractive.

THE CLINICS ARE NOW AVAILABLE ONLINE!

Access your subscription at:
http://www.theclinics.com

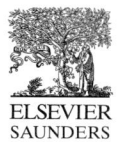

RHEUMATIC
DISEASE CLINICS
OF NORTH AMERICA

ELSEVIER
SAUNDERS

Rheum Dis Clin N Am 31 (2005) xiii–xiv

Preface

Early Rheumatoid Arthritis

For many years, early management of arthritis has been viewed as the ideal approach. However, implementation requires patients to be seen early and treated appropriately at the earliest opportunity. This has been hampered by a number of obstacles. Perhaps the most important one being the fact that referring physicians saw no urgency in identifying appropriate patients because of a lack of evidence that early intervention was effective. Furthermore, it was hard to select the appropriate patients because clinical features did not distinguish self-limiting from persistent disease and there were no diagnostic tests available. Therefore, rather than referring inappropriately, primary care physicians (logically) thought it was more appropriate to watch, wait, and efficiently refer the few patients in whom the disease had manifested itself as rheumatoid arthritis (RA).

In recent years this attitude has changed thanks to evidence that early intervention is the most effective clinical strategy. In this issue of *Rheumatic Disease Clinics of North America*, we review from numerous viewpoints the contemporary management of early RA. In the first article, Drs. Quinn and Cox update the evidence documenting the efficacy of early intervention, providing compelling evidence that patients seen and treated earlier fare better in the short- and long-term. In the second article, Dr. Cush looks at the inertia of primary care referral and how to overcome the obstacles from a primarily American point-of-view, where management of early RA is just one of the issues.

The concept of an evolving early arthritis has emerged, and the importance of an undifferentiated arthritis is now appreciated. Drs. Hitchon, Peschken, Shaikh, and El-Gabalawy discuss the clinical and pathologic features of the very interesting early undifferentiated arthritis population. Patients who have oligo-arthritis (arthritis with involvement of up to four joints) are a neglected subgroup. The article by Drs. Marzo-Ortega, Cawkwell, and Green describes the first clinical trial of oligoarthritis which affects a young population, and note the relatively poor outcome, clinical features, and therapy.

Psoriatic arthritis is the second most common inflammatory disorder in RA and has been enigmatic by definition as it is difficult to differentiate from other forms of arthritis. In its early form, it is poorly described, and inception cohorts

doi:10.1016/j.rdc.2005.10.002   *rheumatic.theclinics.com*

have not been documented. The features of early disease are described comprehensively by Drs. Kane and Pathare in a cohort studied in Ireland.

The cohorts of what might be described as established early RA have been followed for a number of years, and Dr. Young describes their clinical features and an outcome in a wide-ranging review of the area discussing the major long-term studies.

Imaging has been a mainstay of outcome in inflammatory arthritis and radiology has been the gold standard as described by Drs. Boonen and van der Heijde in their article. Meanwhile, new imaging modalities have been developed: of particular interest are the more sensitive and multiplanar modalities such as a three-dimensional MR imaging and ultrasound as described by Drs. Keen, Brown, Wakefield, and Conaghan. Dr. Haugeberg stresses the value of dual energy x-ray absorptiometry. Its precision makes it an extremely valuable diagnostic aid because bone loss of RA is both unique and universal.

It has been the outcome of therapy which has really driven the need and appropriateness of early referral, and appropriate therapy given early has proved much more effective than that given late. The impact of conventional disease-modifying antirheumatic drugs as monotherapy and in combination with various other approaches is described by Drs. Sokka, Hannonen, and Möttönen. The exciting development of biologics applied to early arthritis is described in the article by Drs. de Vries-Bouwstra, Dijkmans, and Breedveld who include the most recent data aiming at biologic-free remission. In the final article, Dr. Quinn highlights the possibilities for altering substantially the population in the circle window of opportunity. Thus this small issue of the *Rheumatic Disease Clinics of North America* moves from theory to practical management.

Paul Emery, MA, MD, FRCP
Academic Unit of Musculoskeletal Disease
Rheumatology and Rehabilitation Research Unit
Chapel Allerton Hospital
Great George Street
Leeds LS1 3EX, UK
E-mail address: p.emery@leeds.ac.uk

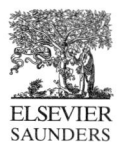ELSEVIER
SAUNDERS

RHEUMATIC
DISEASE CLINICS
OF NORTH AMERICA

Rheum Dis Clin N Am 31 (2005) 575–589

The Evidence for Early Intervention

Mark A. Quinn, MBChB, MRCP*, Sally Cox, BMBS

*Academic Unit of Musculoskeletal Disease, Department of Rheumatology,
Chapel Allerton Hospital, Leeds, UK*

It is believed that rheumatoid arthritis (RA) is the most common, potentially treatable cause of disability in the Western world [1]. A commonsense approach to the management of a persistent, progressive, damaging condition such as RA would seem to be intervention before the onset of damage, at a stage when disease still may be reversible. Such a phase of disease has been described as a "window of opportunity" for intervention [2], but what is the evidence for this?

When does rheumatoid arthritis start?

Immunologic events in RA occur many years before the onset of clinical disease. Rheumatoid factor has been shown in patients years before the onset of symptoms [3]. Similarly, anti–cyclic citrullinated peptide antibodies precede disease by 14 years and precede the detection of rheumatoid factor by an average of 2.8 years [4]. Increases in highly sensitive C-reactive protein (CRP) have been shown before onset of clinical disease in patients with or without serologic abnormalities [5]. When serologic events occur in the presence of the appropriate genetic environment, disease activation would seem even more likely. The risk of developing RA if a patient is positive for anti–cyclic citrullinated peptide and has at least one allele of the shared epitope is increased almost 67-fold [6]. In addition, environmental factors are important, particularly heavy smoking, which is associated with an increased risk of development of seropositive RA [7,8]. These data confirm that the activation of RA is multifactorial with autoimmune

---

* Corresponding author. Academic Unit of Musculoskeletal Disease, Department of Rheumatology, Chapel Allerton Hospital, Chapeltown Road, Leeds, LS7 4SA, UK.

E-mail address: m.quinn@leeds.ac.uk (M.A. Quinn).

0889-857X/05/$ – see front matter
doi:10.1016/j.rdc.2005.07.001   *rheumatic.theclinics.com*

and genetic factors important, most likely in conjunction with appropriate environmental stimuli.

Complementary to the serologic changes detected before clinically manifest disease, imaging and arthroscopy detect synovitis in clinically normal joints. Ultrasound and MRI are able to show the presence of synovitis in patients with early RA in joints with a normal clinical examination [9]. Also in early oligoarthritis, ultrasound has shown subclinical synovitis to be widespread, with 50% of patients having polyarticular disease and the presence of subclinical synovitis correlated with persistence and outcome [10]. Macroscopic and microscopic data from arthroscopy in clinically normal knees of RA patients support these findings, showing significant inflammatory disease [11]. The serologic and imaging data question the sensitivity of clinical examination for detection of low-grade synovitis and timing of true "early" disease. The reality is that by the time a patient presents to a rheumatologist with clinically apparent inflammatory joint disease, immunologic processes and inflammation already are established.

Are rheumatoid arthritis classification criteria useful?

The American College of Rheumatology (ACR) classification criteria for RA were developed to improve homogeneity of patients entered into clinical trials with established disease [12]. It is erroneous to use the criteria for the purpose of diagnosis, especially in the early stages. Patients who satisfy 1987 ACR classification criteria for RA, with very short disease duration, can have a qualitative change in their outcome when treated at presentation, with 50% remission rates after a single dose of corticosteroid with disease of less than 12 weeks' duration [13]. The principal problem is that the very early diagnosis of RA can be difficult because the disease may be indistinguishable from conditions such as postviral arthropathies, early spondyloarthropathy, and other, self-limiting arthritides that may satisfy the 1987 ACR RA criteria [14]. The crucial issue for management of patients with early inflammatory arthritis is initially to establish that it is inflammatory and then to predict persistence. Of the parameters that have

---

Box 1. The Netherlands model to predict persistent (erosive) disease

Symptom duration at first visit
Early morning stiffness for > 60 minutes
Arthritis in > 3 joints
Bilateral compression pain in metatarsophalangeal joints
Anticyclic citrullinated peptide antibody positivity
Erosions on hand or feet x-rays

Table 1
The persistent inflammatory symmetrical arthritis scoring system

Prognostic factor	Score
Rheumatoid factor positive	1
HLA DR1/DR4/DR10	1
C-reactive protein >20 mg/L	1
Female sex	1
HAQ raw score $>4 \leq 11$[a]	1
HAQ raw score >11[a]	2
Total score	7

Abbreviation: HAQ, Health Assessment Questionnaire.
    [a] An HAQ score >3 indicates a poor prognosis.

been examined, symptom duration greater than 12 [13] or 14 [15] weeks seems to be the best single predictor. Symptom duration of at least 12 weeks may be practically more useful for application in future RA diagnostic criteria, as opposed to the 6 weeks currently delineated in the ACR RA classification. The Leiden Early Arthritis Clinic developed a clinical model for prediction of self-limiting arthritis versus a persistent nonerosive or erosive course (Box 1). It incorporated seven parameters and was shown to have a higher discriminative ability than ACR criteria for differentiating between self-limiting and persistent arthritis and between persistent nonerosive and erosive disease [16]. A model for predicting severity in early arthritis also was developed. The persistent inflammatory symmetrical arthritis scoring system combined five parameters, including serology, gender, and baseline function, as indicators of poorer prognosis in early arthritis (Table 1).

What is the importance of early disease?

It already has been established that disease may predate symptoms by many years. For the purposes of clinical trials in early RA, symptom duration of less than 2 years has been the convention, with a shift toward 12 months in recent years. This duration was chosen because, at the end of this period, most patients have incurred significant damage when treated conventionally. Also no prior disease-modifying antirheumatic drug (DMARD) therapy or corticosteroid use is deemed appropriate for optimal data interpretation because these may alter the immunologic and pharmacologic parameters. A case could be made for shorter disease duration, and many groups are now starting to study groups with disease duration less than 12 weeks and asymptomatic, serology-positive groups.

There is considerable evidence that radiographic damage, loss of function [17], and loss of bone mineral density—both axial [18] and peripheral [19,20]— occur early in the disease process. In early RA (< 6 months of symptoms), 40% of patients have erosive disease at presentation [21]. Even with the early arthritis clinic approach, 25% of patients have radiographic erosions at presentation [22].

New imaging techniques show bone changes occur even earlier than was first thought. Bone edema, the MRI precursor to erosions, can be seen in patients after only 4 weeks of symptoms [23]. Ultrasound also can show erosions before they are evident on plain radiography [24].

Another key issue in contemplating the management of a newly diagnosed RA patient is that spontaneous drug-free remission is extremely rare. Remission implies a low disease activity state that if sustained is neither damaging nor disabling. The definition of remission is complex, however, and may not be accurate because it often depends on clinical examination, which, based on imaging studies, is unreliable [9]. Definitions also vary from no active disease on examination to the rigorous ACR remission criteria [25]. The interpretation is confused further by the use of drugs—DMARDs, nonsteroidal anti-inflammatory drugs (NSAIDs), or even simple analgesics. The number of patients whose disease spontaneously remits without therapy is unknown. As evidence accumulates that nontreatment is harmful, it becomes ethically difficult to study untreated patients with active RA. Whichever definition is applied, the prevalence of remission remains low and is inherently different in very early disease compared with established RA [13].

Using the definition of no arthritis on examination and no DMARD therapy for 3 months, only 5% of 258 patients with early RA in primary care entered sustained remission, with or without DMARD therapy, after 2 years' follow-up [26]. Similarly in a study of 183 patients in secondary care, only 7% of patients entered sustained remission over 5 years with routine care, in which remission was defined as four of five of the ACR criteria satisfied with fatigue being excluded [27]. From their results, Harrison et al [26] also concluded that it was not possible to produce a predictive model for remission that would be useful in clinical decision making. Remission in patients with RA is rare and unpredictable at disease outset. It also has been hypothesized that patients with a good prognosis who do well, including patients who enter spontaneous remission, represent a disease that is a separate entity distinguishable from RA by the primary disease site [28]. Spontaneous remission without treatment in patients with established persistent disease may be so rare as to be virtually nonexistent in "true" RA. Conversely, true RA may always be persistent and require aggressive treatment.

What is the evidence to support early intervention?

The level of CRP is used as a surrogate marker of inflammation and progression of radiographic damage [29–31]; loss of function and bone mineral density correlates well with persistent elevation of the CRP. Suppression of CRP results in at least stabilization of the respective parameters [17,18,32,33]. This situation reinforces the paradigm: inflammation $\times$ time = damage [34].

From longitudinal MRI studies in early RA, synovitis seems to precede bone edema and subsequent erosions. Erosions do not occur in the absence of synovitis, and, perhaps more importantly, it has been shown that if synovitis is adequately suppressed, MRI shows reduced bone edema and absence of new bony lesions [35]. It seems that adequate suppression of synovitis prevents progression of bone damage. Previously, radiographic progression has been described despite what seems to be adequate clinical disease suppression [36]. This progression can be explained by (1) the accepted lag time from the time of true damage to radiographically detectable erosions and (2) continued sub-clinical synovitis. MRI research has shown that MRI erosions correlate with radiographic erosions, with a median lag time of 2 years [37].

Not only does damage occur early, but also reversibility of functional loss may be lost with time. Patients treated less than 2 years from disease onset showed a significant improvement in function, using the Health Assessment Questionnaire, after intervention compared with patients treated beyond this time point in a study of 440 patients [38]. In a review of 11 different studies involving 1435 patients, Anderson et al [39] showed that disease duration was paramount in predicting response to DMARD therapy. Of patients, 53% presenting with less than 1 year's disease duration showed a response, whereas later groups (1 to 2 years, 2 to 5 years, 5 to 10 years, and > 10 years) showed diminished responses with time. Similarly, in a study of 448 RA patients, the patients who presented with less than 5 years' disease duration maintained a lower mortality ratio over 21.5 years of follow-up compared with late presenters [40].

Is disease-modifying antirheumatic drug treatment more toxic?

In practical terms, 90% of patients diagnosed with RA are treated with DMARDs within 3 years of diagnosis [1]; most patients eventually are subjected to potential DMARD toxicity. NSAIDs have been compared with DMARDs by calculating a toxicity index derived from symptoms, abnormal laboratory measures, and hospitalizations related to treatment [41,42]. The comparisons show that some commonly used NSAIDs have toxicity indices considerably greater than intramuscular gold and hydroxychloroquine and comparable to methotrexate and azathioprine. In context, DMARD toxicity is no worse than that of long-term NSAID use. From this evidence, delaying use of DMARDs on toxicity grounds is unfounded. In addition, studies looking at any DMARD use versus NSAID or no therapy strongly favor DMARD use with respect to long-term disability index [43] and deformed/damaged joint and radiographic score [44]. Although NSAIDs provide symptom relief in inflammatory arthritis, there is no evidence that they alter disease course.

Immunologic processes precede clinical disease by many years, and sub-clinical disease seems widespread at the time of initial presentation. Damage occurs even earlier than was first thought from data using new imaging modalities, and if inflammation can be adequately suppressed, progression of damage does not occur. When persistence is established, remission occurs more rarely, and withholding DMARDs cannot be justified either for toxicity reasons or for "a watch and wait approach" because most patients are treated regardless of time.

Published studies in early rheumatic arthritis

There are no meta-analyses of therapy in early RA. Trials selected here for review study only patients with disease duration less than 2 years.

Placebo-controlled studies

Evidence shows that long-term, placebo-controlled studies produce unacceptable irreversible damage in the placebo-treated arm [45] and may be unethical. It has been suggested that use of placebo in RA clinical trials is ethical as long as standards of care are maintained [46]. It is now widely believed, however, that the evidence that prolonged exposure to unsuppressed inflammation is damaging is unequivocal, and to expose a patient to this when effective interventions are available remains unethical. As a result, most modern early RA clinical trials use an active comparator arm, usually monotherapy with a conventional DMARD.

In considering the published placebo-controlled studies, sulfasalazine has been shown to improve clinical outcome over 12 months and reduce radiologic damage [21,47]. Hydroxychloroquine also improves clinical outcome, but has not been shown to reduce radiologic damage compared with placebo [48,49].

Delayed introduction of treatment

Other studies have compared early DMARD introduction versus delayed DMARD use. Studies using oral gold have shown clinical benefit and sustained radiologic improvement up to 5 years in favor of early intervention [50]. When use of intramuscular gold was compared at different stages of disease, early use produced the most improvement in functional status [38], and in a separate study using intramuscular gold, a delay in introduction of therapy by 6 months resulted in significant differences in radiographic progression [51]. Van der Heide et al [52] compared DMARD treatment with NSAIDs alone and delayed introduction of DMARDs. All clinically relevant variables were improved at 1 year. No significant difference was detected in radiographic progression; this may have been due to a type 2 statistical error or a larger number of discontinuations in the non–DMARD-treated patients and greater use of corticosteroid in this group [52].

Studies comparing conventional disease-modifying antirheumatic drugs

An increasing number of studies have compared one DMARD with another in an attempt to show greater effectiveness. Sulfasalazine was shown to reduce radiographic progression significantly in a double-blind trial compared with hydroxychloroquine [53] over 48 weeks, but failed to show a significant difference in clinical outcome measures [54]. A comparison of cyclosporine with chloroquine shows a trend toward improved efficacy and similar tolerability with chloroquine [55], and a comparison of cyclosporine with intramuscular gold shows better tolerability and comparable retardation of radiographic progression [56]. When sulfasalazine was compared with intramuscular gold, a trend toward a greater effect on radiographic progression over 12 months was shown. The analysis was not done on an intention-to-treat basis, however, and survival on the drugs at 12 months was 60% and 52% [57]. When methotrexate was compared with intramuscular gold, similar clinical efficacy was shown with no difference in radiographic outcomes, but superior tolerability in favor of methotrexate [58,59]. Van Jaarsveld et al [60] compared different treatment strategies—mild versus potent DMARD therapy with a long lag time versus potent DMARD therapy with short lag time. The potent DMARDs were significantly superior at 12 months according to joint score, remission rates, and radiographic progression, but only radiographic progression maintained significance at 24 months. Methotrexate followed by sulfasalazine seemed to offer the best outcome with tolerability over the other strategies. In established disease, leflunomide has shown similar efficacy and tolerability to sulfasalazine in a cohort of 358 patients (42% <2 years' disease duration, 47% DMARD naive) with a more rapid rate of onset and significantly greater reduction in functional disability ($P < .05$) over 24 weeks [61]. When compared with methotrexate over 52 weeks in 482 patients (38% <2 years' duration, 43% DMARD naive), a similar efficacy and a significant functional improvement in favor of leflunomide was shown [62].

Stenger et al [32] provided further evidence for targeted aggressive treatment. By identifying a high-risk group of early RA patients and treating this group with an aggressive treatment strategy, it was possible to reduce the rate of radiographic progression of this group to that of low-risk patients.

Combination disease-modifying antirheumatic drug therapy studies in early rheumatoid arthritis

With evidence of better efficacy of combination treatment, there has been an increasing trend since the 1990s toward the use of combination therapy in early disease, in the hope of complete suppression of synovitis and reduction in radiographic damage, disability, and deformity. The results on the whole are consistent [63].

Dougados et al [64] and Haagsma et al [65] reported studies looking at the combination of methotrexate and sulfasalazine versus the single components alone. The results showed good tolerability, but failed to show a significant difference in clinical and radiographic variables between the groups, despite a trend to favor the combination arm. In both studies, methotrexate showed similar efficacy to sulfasalazine when used as monotherapy [64,65].

Further evidence for inclusion of corticosteroid in a chosen combination comes from Mottenen et al [66]. Greater remission rates were achieved at 12 months, and a significant reduction in radiographic damage was seen at 24 months in the combination group. The ACR 20 responses were not significantly different between the two groups, however.

The COBRA study group reported a step-down therapeutic approach of sulfasalazine plus methotrexate plus prednisolone versus sulfasalazine alone [67]. Although significant radiographic benefits were seen at 80 weeks, disease activity was comparable in the two groups after the steroid therapy was stopped. There also was a trend toward greater bone density loss in the steroid-treated arm. A cost-effectiveness analysis favored the combination group [68]. Perhaps the most important findings were the long-term radiographic data from this study, which showed significant benefit in terms of damage after 5 years after an initial short aggressive intervention [69]. In an attempt to achieve this in early RA patients with a poor prognosis, the authors have used intra-articular injection of all active joints and aggressive therapy with methotrexate plus cyclosporine versus sulfasalazine and aspiration plus injection of significant joint effusions [70]. Results showed better response, but failed to reach the primary end point for ACR or radiology, although there was a trend toward a lower dropout rate owing to lack of efficacy in the combination group.

More aggressive treatment regimens seem to reduce damage for the duration of suppression of inflammation, but there is no evidence for a qualitative change in the disease mechanisms. Using the oncologic analysis, it is clear that initially aggressive regimens result in initial debulking of disease, improvement in damage, and alteration of the early outcome, yet the disease process continues. A quantitative improvement can be attained, but as yet, the qualitative change in outcome, which had been hoped for, has not been shown. Activity returns when treatment is reduced. Adopting a treatment strategy that aims to suppress inflammation through tight disease control and objective patient assessment statistically can improve disease activity scores, radiographic outcomes, function, and quality of life compared with standard care in the outpatient setting [71].

Role of corticosteroids

The role of corticosteroids is controversial, but they are extremely effective in suppressing cyclooxygenase-2 and cytokines. Corticosteroids also have many uses in the management of RA, including remission induction, maintenance therapy, and bridge and rescue therapy. Corticosteroids have several modes of delivery. The aim is to use the minimum dose necessary for effective outcome. When a low dose of prednisolone (7.5 mg) was added to conventional DMARD therapy over 2 years, a significant reduction in bone damage was obtained [72]. When therapy was blindly stopped and the cohort reanalyzed at 3 years, the rate of radiographic progression in the steroid group was similar to that of the placebo arm [73]. As already mentioned, intra-articular corticosteroids can suppress synovitis effectively in metacarpophalangeal joints as shown by MRI [35]. The early benefits seen in the combination studies that use corticosteroids can be explained by the effect of corticosteroids, which was thought to be lost after treatment withdrawal. The COBRA data [69] imply long-term benefits, however, from early aggressive therapy that includes steroids. Data from a study of very early mild inflammatory arthritis with symptom duration less than 12 weeks suggest a single corticosteroid dose may alter disease persistence and result in remission rates of 50% [13]. Corticosteroids are undoubtedly effective, but are limited in practice by toxicity, which is difficult to quantify. Their optimal role in RA management is yet to be decided, but COBRA and TICORA strategies seem to offer additional benefit over conventional approaches.

New therapies

Tumor necrosis factor (TNF)-α–blocking agents are now available. Studies in early disease are emerging. In a study of 632 patients with active early RA (< 3 years), etanercept showed a significant improvement in clinical outcome when measured using ACR improvement area under the curve, but failed to reach significance when the more accepted and conventional ACR improvement criteria were used versus methotrexate over 12 months [74]. There was a significant reduction in erosion score for the higher dose of etanercept (25 mg) at 6 and 12 months, but there was no significant difference in total radiographic score using the modified Sharp method at 12 months. The greatest benefit was seen in the first 6 months, in which the rapid action of etanercept (25 mg) produced significant improvement in clinical and radiographic measures.

In a subanalysis of early RA patients (< 3 years) from the ATTRACT study [75], in which patients resistant to methotrexate received either methotrexate plus placebo or methotrexate plus infliximab 3 mg or 10 mg/kg for 4 or 8 weeks, significant radiographic improvement was seen in all infliximab-treated patients [76]. Radiographic progression was halted effectively in the infliximab-treated patients. Such inhibition of bone damage has not been shown with existing DMARDs. Subsequently the ASPIRE study group showed clinical and radiographic benefits of combination methotrexate plus infliximab (3 mg or 6 mg/kg) over methotrexate alone in a large cohort of patients with active early RA (< 3 years' duration) [77]. More recently, a placebo-controlled pilot study in early RA patients with a poor prognosis using infliximab and methotrexate versus methotrexate alone showed significant differences in functional outcome, quality of life, and MRI erosion scores at 12 months [78]. After withdrawal of the study drug (either infliximab or placebo) at 12 months and a further 12 months of observation, no patient showing a response to infliximab had flare of their disease requiring additional DMARD, and median disease activity score (DAS 28) was maintained at remission levels. Even more important, functional and quality-of-life differences were attained early and remained at 2 years' follow-up. This study using infliximab as induction therapy has shown that early use of anti-TNF-α can produce a sustained benefit. These data qualitatively differ from the studies of conventional DMARDs, in which structural damage is prevented, but patient-based assessments are not improved.

Clinical and radiologic outcomes of four different treatment strategies in patients with active RA of less than 2 years' duration were assessed in a randomized controlled study [79]. A total of 508 patients were allocated to (1) sequential DMARD therapy, (2) step-up combination therapy, (3) initial combination DMARD with tapered high-dose prednisolone, or (4) methotrexate therapy in conjunction with infliximab. Initial combination therapy with steroid or infliximab showed superior outcome at 1 year in terms of function and radiologic damage.

Use of TNF-α antagonists combined with methotrexate has been shown to be effective in management of early RA. Do these agents offer additional advantage in combination, or are they effective as monotherapy? This question was addressed in the PREMIER study [80]. Methotrexate-naive patients with recent-onset RA were randomized to receive adalimumab, 40 mg, plus methotrexate (escalating dose to 20 mg), or adalimumab or methotrexate alone with the primary end point being ACR 50 and change in total Sharpe Score at 52 weeks. Combination therapy was found to be superior to single-therapy groups in clinical outcomes (ACR 20/50/70, DAS 28, and Health Assessment Questionnaire) at 52 and 104 weeks. Adalimumab plus methotrexate induced remission in 50% of patients at 2 years (DAS 28 < 2.6). Although there was no clinically significant difference in ACR 50 between the single-therapy groups, there was a statistically significant difference in favor of adalimumab in terms of radiographic progression over methotrexate.

Discussion

The benefit of early treatment in RA is supported by published data. Properly conducted studies, with most currently used DMARDs, show clinical improvement and retardation of radiographic damage, although evidence suggests x-ray changes are insensitive and lag considerably behind inflammatory activity [14]. Studies using newer techniques of joint assessment, such as MRI and ultrasound, have shown greater sensitivity and a close temporal correlation with inflammatory activity and damage progression.

Although it is straightforward to show the benefits of early intervention and suppression of inflammation, how best to achieve this is more difficult to assess. There are several inherent difficulties. Corticosteroids have a profound and dramatic early effect when used in therapeutic regimens, yet toxicity generally occurs late. RA itself is a heterogeneous condition, and so is the response of the patient to therapy. What conclusions can be made?

Multiple treatment strategies have been tried: step-up therapy, step-down therapy, bridge therapy, combination therapy, and monotherapy in addition to several variants. No strategy has been proved to be consistently better than another for all patients. A significant factor is the high proportion of good responders to monotherapy alone, who are not improved further by complex therapeutic regimens and for whom the additional cost of extra therapy cannot be justified [58]. The same effect means that at present there is insufficient evidence to recommend routine first-line use of biologic agents. The therapeutic regimen currently being assessed by the authors' unit involves routine use of first-line monotherapy. Poor responders are identified early to limit the development of irreversible damage. Such patients are targeted with escalating combination therapy with continued poor responders receiving biologic agents. The priority for treatment should be rapid and sustained suppression of inflammation.

Data presented are for the most part from randomized trials in which use of adjunct intra-articular, intramuscular, or oral corticosteroid therapy is restricted, and this does not reflect true general rheumatology practice. Effectiveness studies of monotherapy and combination therapy with judicious use of adjunct corticosteroids compared with the new biologic agents are required. The availability of these agents has had a major impact on the management of established RA with marked improvement in quality of life and conventional disease activity measures. It is likely that in determining future optimal therapeutic regimens for early RA, health economic issues will dominate [66].

References

[1] Emery P, Salmon M. Early rheumatoid arthritis: time to aim for remission? Ann Rheum Dis 1995;54:944–7.

[2] Quinn MA, Emery P. Window of opportunity in early rheumatoid arthritis: possibility of altering the disease process with early intervention. Clin Exp Rheum 2003;21(Suppl 31):S154–7.

[3] Aho K, Heliövaara M, Maatela J, et al. Rheumatoid factors antedating clinical rheumatoid arthritis. J Rheumatol 1991;18:1282–4.

[4] Nielen MJ, van Schaardenburg D, Reesink HW, et al. Specific autoantibodies precede the symptoms of rheumatoid arthritis: a study of serial measurements in blood donors. Arthritis Rheum 2004;50:380–6.

[5] Nielen MJ, van Schaardenburg D, Reesink HW, et al. Increased levels of C-reactive protein in serum from blood donors before the onset of rheumatoid arthritis. Arthritis Rheum 2004;50: 2423–7.

[6] Berglin E, Padyukov L, Sundin U, et al. A combination of autoantibodies to cyclic citrullinated peptide (CCP) and HLA DRB-1 locus antigens is strongly associated with future onset of rheumatoid arthritis. Arthritis Res Ther 2004;6:R303–8.

[7] Padyukov L, Silva C, Stolt P, et al. A gene-environment interaction between smoking and shared epitope genes in HLA-DR provides a high risk of seropositive rheumatoid arthritis. Arthritis Rheum 2004;50:3085–92.

[8] Stolt P, Bengtsson C, Nordmark B, et al. Quantification of the influence of cigarette smoking on the rheumatoid arthritis: results from a population based case-control, using incident cases. Ann Rheum Dis 2003;62:835–41.

[9] Conaghan PG, Wakefield RJ, O'Connor P, et al. MCPJ assessment in early RA: a comparison between x-ray, MRI, high-resolution ultrasound and clinical examination. Arthritis Rheum 1998;41(Suppl):S246.

[10] Wakefield RJ, Green MJ, Gibbon WW, et al. High resolution ultrasound defined subclinical synovitis—a predictor of outcome in early oligoarthritis? Arthritis Rheum 1998;41(Suppl):S246.

[11] Kraan MC, Versendaal H, Jonker M, et al. Asymptomatic synovitis precedes clinically manifest arthritis. Arthritis Rheum 1998;41:1481–8.

[12] Arnett FC, Edworthy SM, Bloch DA, et al. The American Rheumatism Association 1987 revised criteria for the classification of rheumatoid arthritis. Arthritis Rheum 1988;31:315–24.

[13] Green M, Marzo-Ortega H, McGonagle D, et al. Persistence of mild, early inflammatory arthritis: the importance of disease duration, rheumatoid factor and the shared epitope. Arthritis Rheum 1999;42:2184–8.

[14] Calin A, Marks S. The case against sero-negative rheumatoid arthritis. Am J Med 1981;70: 992–4.

[15] Tunn EJ, Bacon PA. Differentiating persistent from self-limiting symmetrical synovitis in an early arthritis clinic. Br J Rheum 1993;32:97–103.

[16] Visser H, Cessie S, Vos K, et al. How to diagnose rheumatoid arthritis early: a prediction model for persistent (erosive) arthritis. Arthritis Rheum 2002;46:357–65.

[17] Devlin J, Gough A, Huissoon A, et al. The acute phase and function in early RA: CRP levels correlate with functional outcome. J Rheumatol 1997;24:9–13.

[18] Gough AK, Lilley J, Eyre S, et al. Generalised bone loss in patients with early RA occurs early and relates to disease activity. Lancet 1994;344:23–7.

[19] Deodhar A, Brabyn J, Jones PW, et al. Longitudinal study of hand bone densitometry in rheumatoid arthritis. Arthritis Rheum 1995;38:1204–10.

[20] Devlin J, Lilley J, Gough A, et al. Clinical associations with DXA measurement of hand bone mass in rheumatoid arthritis. Br J Rheumatol 1996;35:1256–62.

[21] Hannonen P, Mottenen T, Hakola M, Oka M. Sulfasalazine in early rheumatoid arthritis: a 48 week double-blind, prospective, placebo-controlled study. Arthritis Rheum 1993;36:1501–9.

[22] Van der Horst-Bruinsma I, Speyer I, Visser H, et al. Diagnosis and course of early-onset arthritis: results of a special early arthritis clinic compared to routine patient care. Br J Rheumatol 1998; 37:1084–8.

[23] McGonagle D, Conaghan PG, O'Connor P, et al. The relationship between synovitis and bone changes in early untreated rheumatoid arthritis. Arthritis Rheum 1999;42:1706–11.

[24] Wakefield RJ, McGonagle D, Green MJ, et al. A comparison of high resolution sonography with MRI and conventional radiography for the detection of erosions in early rheumatoid arthritis. Br J Rheumatol 1998;37(Suppl):105.

[25] Pinals RS, Masi AT, Larsen RA. Preliminary criteria for clinical remission in rheumatoid arthritis. Arthritis Rheum 1981;24:1138–42.

[26] Harrison BJ, Symmons DPM, Brennan P, et al. Natural remission in inflammatory polyarthritis: issues of definition and prediction. Br J Rheumatol 1996;35:1096–100.

[27] Eberhardt K, Fex E. Clinical course and remission rate in patients with early rheumatoid arthritis: relationship to outcome after 5 years. Br J Rheumatol 1998;37:1324–9.

[28] McGonagle D, Gibbon WW, O'Connor P, et al. An anatomical explanation for good prognosis rheumatoid arthritis. Lancet 1999;353:123–4.

[29] Van Leeuwen MA, Van Rijswijk MH, Sluiter WJ, et al. Individual relationship between progression of radiological damage and the acute phase response in early rheumatoid arthritis: towards development of a decision support system. J Rheumatol 1997;24:20–7.

[30] Fex E, Eberhardt K, Saxne T. Tissue derived macromolecules and markers of inflammation in serum in early rheumatoid arthritis: relationship to development of joint destruction in hands and feet. Br J Rheumatol 1997;36:1161–5.

[31] Amos RA, Constable TJ, Crockson RA, et al. Rheumatoid arthritis: relationship of C-reactive protein and erythrocyte sedimentation rates and radiographic change. BMJ 1977;1:195–7.

[32] Stenger AAME, Van Leuewen MA, Houtman PM, et al. Early effective suppression of inflammation in rheumatoid arthritis reduces radiographic progression. Br J Rheumatol 1998; 37:1157–63.

[33] Dawes PT, Fowler PD, Clarke S, et al. Rheumatoid arthritis: treatment which controls the C-reactive protein and erythrocyte sedimentation rate reduces radiological progression. Br J Rheumatol 1986;25:44–9.

[34] Emery P. The optimal management of early rheumatoid arthritis: the key to preventing disability. Br J Rheumatol 1994;33:765–8.

[35] Conaghan PG, O'Connor P, McGonagle D, et al. Elucidation of the relationship between synovitis and bone damage: a randomized magnetic resonance imaging study of individual joints in patients with early rheumatoid arthritis. Arthritis Rheum 2003;48:64–71.

[36] Mulherin D, Fitzgerald O, Bresnihan B. Clinical improvement and radiological deterioration in rheumatoid arthritis: evidence that the pathogenesis of synovial inflammation and articular damage may differ. Br J Rheumatol 1996;35:1263–8.

[37] Østergaard M, Hansen M, Stoltenberg M, et al. New radiographic bone erosions in the wrists of patients with rheumatoid arthritis are detectable with magnetic resonance imaging a median of two years earlier. Arthritis Rheum 2003;48:2128–31.

[38] Munro R, Hampson R, McEntergart A, et al. Improved functional outcome in patients with early rheumatoid arthritis treated with intramuscular gold: results of a five year prospective study. Ann Rheum Dis 1998;57:88–93.

[39] Anderson JJ, Wells G, Verhoeven AC, Felson DT. Factors predicting response to treatment in rheumatoid arthritis: the importance of disease duration. Arthritis Rheum 2000;43:22–9.

[40] Symmons D, Jones MA, Scott DL, Prior P. Long term mortality outcome in patients with rheumatoid arthritis: early presenters continue to do well. J Rheumatol 1998;25:1072–7.

[41] Fries JF, Williams CA, Bloch DA. The relative toxicity of non-steroidal antiinflammatory drugs. Arthritis Rheum 1991;34:1353–60.

[42] Fries JF, Williams CA, Ramey D, Bloch DA. The relative toxicity of disease-modifying anti-rheumatic drugs. Arthritis Rheum 1993;36:297–306.

[43] Fries J, Williams CA, Morfield D, et al. Reduction in long-term disability in patients with rheumatoid arthritis by disease-modifying antirheumatic drug-based treatment strategies. Arthritis Rheum 1996;39:616–22.

[44] Abu-Shakra M, Toker R, Flusser D, et al. Clinical and radiographic outcomes of rheumatoid arthritis patients not treated with disease modifying drugs. Arthritis Rheum 1998;41:1190–5.

[45] Stein CM, Pincus T. Placebo-controlled studies in rheumatoid arthritis: ethical issues. Lancet 1999;353:400–3.

[46] Schwieterman WD. FDA perspective on anti-TNF treatments. Ann Rheum Dis 1999;58:190–1.

[47] The Australian Multicentre clinical trial group. Sulfasalazine in early RA. J Rheumatol 1992;19:1672–7.

[48] Davis MJ, Dawes PT, Fowler PD, et al. Should disease modifying drugs be used in mild rheumatoid arthritis? Br J Rheumatol 1991;30:451–4.

[49] The HERA study group. A randomised trial of hydroxychloroquine in early rheumatoid arthritis: the HERA study. Am J Med 1995;98:156–68.

[50] Egsmose C, Lund B, Borg G, et al. Patients with early arthritis benefit from early 2nd line therapy: 5 year follow-up of a prospective double blind placebo controlled study. J Rheumatol 1995;22:2208–13.

[51] Buckland-Wright JC, Clarke GS, Chikanza IC, Grahame R. Quantitative microfocal radiography detects changes in erosion area in patients with early rheumatoid arthritis treated with myocrisine. J Rheumatol 1993;20:243–7.

[52] Van der Heide A, Jacobs JWG, Bijlsma JWJ, et al. The effectiveness of early treatment with 'second-line' anti-rheumatic drugs: a randomised controlled trial. Ann Intern Med 1996;124:699–707.

[53] Van der Heijde DM, Van Riel PL, Nuver-Zwart IH, et al. Effects of hydroxychloroquine and sulphasalazine on progression of joint damage in rheumatoid arthritis. Lancet 1989;1:1036–8.

[54] Nuver-Zwart IH, Van Riel PLCM, Van de Putte LBA, Gribnau FWJ. A double blind comparative study of sulphasalazine and hydroxychloroquine in rheumatoid arthritis: evidence of an earlier effect of sulphasalazine. Ann Rheum Dis 1989;48:389–95.

[55] Van den Borne BE, Landewe RB, The HS, et al. Low dose cyclosporin in early rheumatoid arthritis: effective and safe after two years of therapy when compared to chloroquine. Scand J Rheumatol 1996;25:307–16.

[56] Zeidler HK, Kvien TK, Hannonen P, et al. Progression of joint damage in early active severe rheumatoid arthritis during eighteen months of treatment: comparison of low dose cyclosporin and parenteral gold. Br J Rheumatol 1998;37:874–82.

[57] Peltomaa R, Paimela L, Helve T, Leirisalo-Repo M. Comparison of intramuscular gold and sulphasalazine in the treatment of early rheumatoid arthritis: a one year prospective study. Scand J Rheumatol 1995;24:330–5.

[58] Menninger H, Herborn G, Sander O, et al. A 36 month comparative trial of methotrexate and gold sodium thiomalate in the treatment of early active and erosive rheumatoid arthritis. Br J Rheumatol 1998;37:1060–8.

[59] Rau R, Herborn G, Karger T, et al. Progression in early erosive rheumatoid arthritis: 12 month results from a randomised controlled trial comparing methotrexate and gold sodium thiomalate. Br J Rheumatol 1998;37:1220–6.

[60] Van Jaarsveld CHM, Jacobs JWG, van der Veen MJ, et al. Aggressive treatment in early rheumatoid arthritis: a randomised controlled trial. Ann Rheum Dis 2000;59:468–77.

[61] Smolen JS, Kalden JK, Scott DL, et al. Efficacy and safety of leflunomide compared with placebo and sulphasalazine in active rheumatoid arthritis: a double-blind, randomised, multicentre trial. Lancet 1999;353:259–66.

[62] Strand V, Cohen S, Schiff M, et al for the Leflunomide Rheumatoid Arthritis investigators group. Treatment of active rheumatoid arthritis with leflunomide compared with placebo and methotrexate. Arch Intern Med 1999;159:2542–50.

[63] Verhoeven AC, Boers M, Tugwell P, et al. Combination therapy in rheumatoid arthritis: updated systematic review. Br J Rheumatol 1998;37:612–9.

[64] Dougados M, Combe B, Cantagrel A, et al. Combination therapy in early rheumatoid arthritis: a randomised, controlled, double blind 52 week clinical trial of sulphasalazine and methotrexate compared with the single components. Ann Rheum Dis 1999;58:220–5.

[65] Haagsma CJ, Van Riel PLCM, De Jong AJL, Van de Putte LBA. Combination of sulphasalazine and methotrexate versus the single components in early rheumatoid arthritis: a randomised, controlled, double-blind, 52 week clinical trial. Br J Rheumatol 1997;36:1082–8.

[66] Mottenen T, Hannonen P, Leirisalo-Repo M, et al. Comparison of combination therapy with single drug-therapy in early rheumatoid arthritis: a randomised trial. Lancet 1999;353:1568–73.

[67] Boers M, Verhoeven AC, Markusse HM, et al. Randomised comparison of combined step-down prednisolone, methotrexate and sulphasalazine with sulphasalazine alone in early rheumatoid arthritis. Lancet 1997;350:309–18.

[68] Verhoeven AC, Bibo JC, Boers M, et al for the COBRA trial group. Cost-effectiveness and cost-utility of combination therapy in early rheumatoid arthritis: randomized comparison of combined step-down prednisolone, methotrexate and sulphasalazine with sulphasalazine alone. Br J Rheumatol 1998;37:1102–9.

[69] Landewe RB, Boers M, Verhoeven AC, et al. COBRA combination therapy in patients with early rheumatoid arthritis: long-term structural benefits of a brief intervention. Arthritis Rheum 2002; 46:347–56.

[70] Proudman S, Conaghan P, Richardson C, et al. Treatment of poor prognosis early rheumatoid arthritis a randomised study of methotrexate, cyclosporin A and intraarticular corticosteroids compared with sulphasalazine alone. Arthritis Rheum 2000;43:1809–19.

[71] Grigor C, Capell H, Stirling A, et al. Effect of a treatment strategy of tight control for rheumatoid arthritis (the TICORA study): a single-blind randomised study. Lancet 2004;364:263–9.

[72] Kirwan JR and the ARC Low dose glucocorticoid study group. The effect of glucocorticoids on joint destruction in rheumatoid arthritis. N Engl J Med 1995;333:142–6.

[73] Hickling P, Jacoby RK, Kirwan JR and the Arthritis and Rheumatism Council low dose glucocorticosteroid group. Joint destruction after glucocorticoids are withdrawn in early rheumatoid arthritis. Br J Rheum 1998;37:930–6.

[74] Bathon JM, Martin RW, Fleischmann RM, et al. A comparison of etanercept and methotrexate in patients with early rheumatoid arthritis. N Engl J Med 2000;343:1586–93.

[75] Lipsky PE, van der Heijde DMFM, St. Clair EW, et al. Infliximab and methotrexate in the treatment of rheumatoid arthritis. N Engl J Med 2000;343:1594–602.

[76] Breedveld FC, Emery P, Keystone E, et al. Infliximab in active early rheumatoid arthritis. Ann Rheum Dis 2004;63:149–55.

[77] St Clair EW, van der Heijde DM, Smolen JS, et al. Combination of infliximab and methotrextae therapy for early rheumatoid arthritis: a randomised controlled trial. Arthritis Rheum 2004; 50:3432–43.

[78] Quinn MA, Conaghan PG, Greenstein A, et al. Very early infliximab in addition to methotrexate in early poor prognosis rheumatoid arthritis reduces MRI synovitis and damage with
sustained benefit after infliximab withdrawal: results from a double blind placebo-controlled
trial. Arthritis Rheum 2005;52:27–35.
[79] De Vries-Bouwstra JK, Goekoop-Ruiterman YPM, van Zeben D, et al. A comparison of clinical
and radiological outcomes of four treatment strategies for early rheumatoid arthritis: results of the
BEST trial. Ann Rheum Dis 2004;63(Suppl):58.
[80] Breedveld FC, Kavanaugh A, Cohen S, et al. Early treatment of rheumatoid arthritis with
adalimumab plus methotrexate versus adalimumab alone or methotrexate alone: the PREMIER
study. Arthritis Rheum 2004;50:4096–7.

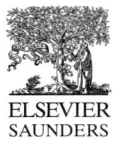

ELSEVIER
SAUNDERS

RHEUMATIC
DISEASE CLINICS
OF NORTH AMERICA

Rheum Dis Clin N Am 31 (2005) 591–604

Remodeling a Rheumatology Practice to Facilitate Early Referral

John J. Cush, MD*

Department of Rheumatology and Clinical Immunology, Presbyterian Hospital of Dallas, Dallas, TX, USA

The belief in early diagnosis and aggressive treatment of rheumatoid arthritis (RA) has become a cornerstone for rheumatologists worldwide [1,2]. Although the benefits seem inherently obvious, this paradigm shift has resulted from decades of work showing that earlier diagnosis and optimal use of drug therapy can yield long-term patient benefits. Conversely, patients deprived of early intervention uniformly show poor functional, morbid, and mortal outcomes [3–5]. Delays in starting disease-modifying antirheumatic drug (DMARD) therapy, even delays of 3 to 4 months, can have disappointing downstream effects on radiographic, functional and work outcomes [3–6]. This article focuses on current efforts in North America to revise medical practice and patient referral to afford early arthritis patients a chance at a timely diagnosis and expert treatment.

Limited data on earlier rheumatoid arthritis referral

There is a paucity of documentation on the presumed trend in earlier patient referral to rheumatologists. Nonetheless, there are few reports of declining referral times from primary care physicians (PCPs) to rheumatology specialty care and the earlier use of DMARD therapies by rheumatologists. In 1994, Chan and colleagues [7] reported their 1987–1990 experience of a Massachusetts managed care system and the referral of newly diagnosed RA patients. Although

Dr. Cush currently is an investigator for Abbott, Amgen, Genetech, and the National Institutes of Health and a consultant for Abbott, Amgen, Wyeth, Centocor, and Regeneron.

* Department of Rheumatology and Clinical Immunology, Presbyterian Hospital of Dallas, 8200 Walnut Hill Lane, Dallas, TX 75231-4496.

E-mail address: jackcush@texashealth.org

the median time from symptom onset to first physician encounter was only 4 weeks, the median average time to a diagnosis of RA was 36 weeks (range 4 weeks to 10 years). The diagnosis was made by the PCP only 12% of the time, and the lag time from first medical encounter to rheumatology referral was 1 to 74 weeks (median 8 weeks). In Glasgow, researchers described the evolution of referral lag times in 198 consecutive newly diagnosed RA patients between 1980 and 1997 [8]. Over this time frame, the lag time from symptom onset to general practitioner referral significantly decreased from a mean of 21 months to 4 months. The lag time to DMARD initiation also decreased from 32 months to 1 month. Lastly, the number of patients starting DMARD therapy within the first 6 months increased from 5% before 1994 to 44% by 1997. These data suggest that patients may be diagnosed earlier and given DMARDs in a timely manner. In contrast, in 2000, Hernandez-Garcia and colleagues [9] noted that of the 527 new RA patients seen in their rheumatology clinics, it took nearly 17 months for patients to be referred to a rheumatologist. Nonetheless, it took only an average of 2 months for rheumatologists to initiate DMARD therapy in these newly diagnosed RA patients.

Need for early referral in North America

In most North American rheumatology practices, *very early RA* (defined as symptom duration <12 weeks) and *early RA* (defined as symptom duration < 24 weeks) patients rarely are seen as new patient encounters. Reliable, population-based data that document health care use by new-onset arthritis or RA patients are unavailable. Most RA patients entering a North American rheumatology practice already have a diagnosis of RA, have years of symptoms, had previous serologic tests, and have had multiple attempts at drug therapy (including corticosteroids and immunosuppressive agents).

Why is the early RA patient so rarely seen? Either such patients are scarce, or there may be significant impediments to access or consultation. Barriers that hinder expedient and early patient referral are numerous and include the shortfall in number of practicing rheumatologists, deficient PCP skills in musculoskeletal diagnosis, overreliance on laboratory diagnostics, erroneous referral to other practitioners (eg, orthopedists, physiatrists, podiatrists), patient reluctance to seek medical attention for new and nonlimiting joint symptoms, lack of health care benefits, and the availability of over-the-counter medications. Most rheumatologists believe they are not the problem, but instead individually are making efforts to resolve this problem. Although they admit to hectic schedules and long wait times for consultation (usually 8–24 weeks) (M. Schiff, unpublished abstract: "Survey or rheumatology practices"), rheumatologists believe they can accommodate urgent referrals simply with a call from their PCP colleagues. These well-intentioned and informal policies are not well described or promoted, however. Rapid or urgent referrals that require physician-to-physician phone requests, transfer of medical records and tests, and insurance preapprovals are, by their nature, a deterrent to most rheumatology referrals. Few rheumatologists have altered their practices by committing to dedicated early arthritis time slots or an early arthritis clinic (EAC). Most rheumatologists believe that the task of dedicating a clinic to "early arthritis" would be burdensome and costly in lost time or revenue. Many agree that such early arthritis activities are best suited for academic and research sites. Rheumatologists also have apprehensions about efforts to educate PCPs about early RA and when to refer. The assumption that most patients in need will find their way to appropriate care is optimistic and without evidence. Direct-to-consumer advertising targeting RA and the need for referral (for new medicines) has been pervasive in the United States and may increase population awareness, but it has had little or no effect on the care of patients with undiagnosed RA or new-onset polyarthritis.

Documentation of this unmet need is lacking. There are population-based statistics, however, on the incidence rates for inflammatory arthritis and RA. In one study, the incidence of inflammatory arthritis was 115 cases per 100,000 persons per year [10]. By contrast, the incidence of RA from many studies ranges from 15 to 40 new cases per 100,000 persons per year [11,12]. A large city with a population of 1 million should expect 200 to 350 new cases of RA each year. Thus, in the next 12 months, new-onset RA will afflict more than 7500 Canadians and more than 75,000 Americans. Only a few of these patients will be cared for by rheumatologists. The average rheumatologist cares for 250 to 500 RA patients and usually sees 5 to 10 new-onset RA (disease duration <12 months) patients each year. The current number of practicing rheumatologists in Canada and the United States would allow for these new patients to be seen. In the United States, less than 4000 practicing rheumatologists would have to take in 17 to 23 new RA patients each per year to manage the nation's 75,000 cases.

Reasons to refer early rheumatoid arthritis patients

Considerable research and effort in the 1990s have documented the success of novel programs focused on patients with early inflammatory arthritis or early RA. This body of work has given credence to possibility that an early RA diagnosis affords each patient with a significant advantage such that appropriate early interventions can yield significant long-term benefits [1–6,13,14]. EACs have been in place for more than a decade in Austria, Germany, Finland, France, The Netherlands, and the United Kingdom, with resultant activities that have influenced patient care and physicians' understanding of incipient or early RA. These EACs have been a prime forum for novel research on RA outcomes, prognostic factors, and novel therapeutics. The success of these EACs has stirred the interest of North American rheumatologists, but has not caused a remodeling of their current practices. In addition, the predicted rheumatology manpower shortages in the next 2 decades would substantially increase the workload burden for North American rheumatologists. The American College of Rheumatology has predicted that by 2020, the number of U.S. rheumatologists will decline by nearly 20%, at a time when an aging U.S. population will increase the number of patients with arthritis to more than 100 million persons [15]. Currently, there is no plan to meet this societal burden. The number of trainees going into rheumatology is low. A partial answer to this dilemma is for the practicing rheumatologist not to work harder, but instead to work smarter by focusing on patients who would benefit most from their expertise.

Many lines of evidence favor the need to promote rapid referral, early diagnosis, and aggressive treatment. This evidence (discussed in detail in other articles in this issue) briefly includes the following:

- Hallert and colleagues [16] showed that 63% of early RA patients experience work disability during the first year, which substantially increased the cost of care.
- Health Assessment Questionnaire scores in the first year have been shown to predict future loss of productivity and disability [17].
- Many studies have documented histologic inflammation, serologic abnormalities (rheumatoid factor [RF] and cyclic citrullinated peptide antibody [CCP] antibodies), and markers of bone turnover before or soon after the onset of disease [18,19]. It is not surprising that 15% to 25% of patients have erosions at presentation, and that erosive disease occurs in more than 70% of patients in the first 2 years [20].
- There are now reliable clinical and laboratory predictors of a more aggressive course and of patients who may benefit from prompt diagnosis and early aggressive therapies.
- Less than 5% of RA patients achieve true remission [21].
- Newer and more aggressive combination DMARD and biologic regimens have yet to be applied to early RA patients outside of clinical trials [22–24].

The introduction of new DMARDs (methotrexate, cyclosporine, leflunomide) and biologics (tumor necrosis factor [TNF]-α inhibitors, interleukin-1 inhibitors, monoclonal antibodies) has changed the lives of many RA patients dramatically in the last 2 decades [25]. Despite these advances, most RA patients are still not in remission. It is estimated that 15% to 20% of RA patients in the United States (<10% in Canada) are currently receiving TNF-α inhibitors, and that nearly 80% of all TNF-α inhibitor prescriptions are written by only 20% of rheumatologists. These data attest to the therapeutic conservatism of most North American rheumatologists. Although drugs have changed dramatically, rheumatologists have not. This conservatism has entrenched treatment paradigms and may take years to decades to change. Similarly, changes in patient referral and intake would be difficult to implement unless rheumatologists change to meet this demand. Although all rheumatologists strongly advocate for earliest possible diagnosis of RA and the most aggressive treatments possible, few North Americans employ aggressive therapies (other than methotrexate or hydroxychloroquine) in early RA, and even fewer have revised their clinical practice to facilitate the optimal care of these patients.

Survey of North American rheumatologists

A survey was conducted of rheumatologists from the United States and Canada known to have an interest in establishing an EAC or to have a currently existing EAC (see Acknowledgments). The purpose of this survey was to describe the types of EAC clinics in existence, the tools required for initiation, and how each clinic performs. Additionally, this panel was presented with a new-onset patient vignette and asked to rank available therapeutic options. This survey was initiated by e-mail invitation, and respondents were invited to participate in an online survey. Each rheumatologist was allowed one response, and each was asked to provide the names of others in their region or country who also may provide input. Overall, 27 individuals from the United States (two thirds) and Canada (one third) were e-mailed surveys, and 23 (85%) responded to all or some of the questions (Table 1).

Most respondents were men, in practice for 10 to 25 years (>70%), and currently employed at academic centers (70%) or in group/solo practices (30%). The primary motivation for establishing an EAC was to expand research/clinical trials (70%) or recent review of the early arthritis medical literature (55%). Despite an expressed EAC interest, only 52% currently were operating an active EAC, another 22% were in the planning stages, 9% previously ran a clinic, and 17% did not yet have an EAC [4]. Although 15% of EACs were devoted to early RA only, the remaining 85% focused on either early undiagnosed or inflammatory arthritis. Promotional efforts largely were restricted to letters to PCPs (68%), PCP-directed education (32%), and hospital publications (26%). Only a few EACs (<16%) employed public relations, local signs, newspaper articles, press releases, letters to patients, Internet web pages, or dedicated phone lines. All required referrals for early arthritis consultation, either from a physician (65%) or from another health care provider (35%). Entry required symptoms of less than 12 months' duration in 90%, and one clinic required symptoms of less than 3 months' duration. EACs meet at least weekly for 79% of respondents and usually are staffed by rheumatologists (90%), rheumatology fellows (35%), nurse practitioners or physician assistants (40%), or study coordinators (30%). These clinics see an average of 5.5 patients (median 4, range 1–25) per clinic. The EAC appointment wait time was less than 2 weeks in 58% of patients, and all patients were seen within 4 weeks. Most centers projected that they would see an average of 332 patients (range 20–1200) in the next 12 months. Patients were screened for eligibility using a PCP referral form (80%), limits on joint symptom duration (45%), chart review (30%), telephone interview (25%), or a minimum number of swollen joints (20%). At intake, most patients underwent testing for serum RF, erythrocyte sedimentation rate (ESR), C-reactive protein (CRP), and anti-CCP antibody. Half of patients received radiographs, but only a few were routinely tested for hepatitis, parvovirus B19, or *Chlamydia,* and a few received ultrasound or MRI. Most respondents collected a variety of outcome measures, including tender and swollen joint counts, functional surveys (eg, Health Assessment Questionnaire), ESR or CRP, RF, CCP, and radiographs. One in five centers was dedicated to serial MRI or ultrasound, and

Table 1
Survey of North American rheumatology early arthritis clinics

Criteria	Percentage (N = 23)
Requires referral by physician or HCP	100
Limitations on symptom duration for entry	
<12 wk	5
<6 mo	25
<12 mo	60
<24 mo	10
Requirement(s) for EAC eligibility	
PCP referral form	80
Specified limits on symptom duration	45
Minimal number of swollen joints	20
Telephone screening	25
Chart review	30
Patient questionnaire	5
NP or PA screening clinic visit	5
EAC frequency	
Daily	21
Twice weekly	11
Weekly	47
Biweekly	21
Routine EAC diagnostic testing	
Erythrocyte sedimentation rate	95
Rheumatoid factor	95
C-reactive protein	90
Cyclic citrullinated peptide antibody	75
Antinuclear antibody	75
Radiographs	50
Hepatitis B and C serologies	25
Parvovirus B19 serology	20
Ultrasound	25
MRI	10
EAC start-up funds	
None	29
$20,000–50,000	41
$60,000–90,000	18
>$200,000	12

Abbreviations: EAC, early arthritis clinic; HCP, health care provider; MRI magnetic resonance imaging; NP nurse practitioner; PA physician assistant.

15% were involved in synovial fluid or tissue collection. One center routinely testing for the shared epitope. Although no startup funds were needed in 29% of centers, 58% required $20,000 to 90,000 to launch their EAC. When asked how their EAC efforts were received locally, 83% of patients and 61% of PCPs were either positive or enthusiastic; 28% of PCPs were equivocal or disinterested.

Table 2
Survey of early arthritis clinics specialists on management of a very early arthritis patient

Agent	N = 20			
	1st choice	2nd choice	3rd choice	4th choice
Another NSAID	2	—	1	—
Low-dose prednisone	6	4	1	3
Intra-articular steroid	2	3	—	—
Methotrexate	6	5	4	1
Sulfasalazine	—	2	—	2
Hydroxychloroquine	3	2	1	—
TNF-α inhibitor	—	—	2	1
Combination DMARDs	1	3	5	1
Methotrexate + TNF-α inhibitor	—	—	2	3
Clinical trial for early arthritis	1	1	2	3

Vignette: an early arthritis patient presents with 8 weeks of symptoms, uncontrolled by high-dose NSAIDs. The patient has 60 minutes of morning stiffness, four tender and three swollen typical hand joints. Laboratory tests are unavailable. What order of drugs do you prefer to add in the next 6 months?

Although the respondents were consistent with regard to the startup, conduct, and outcome measures in their EAC, they differed in their approach to treatment of newly undiagnosed early inflammatory arthritis patients. Each respondent was presented with a fictional early arthritis clinical vignette (Table 2) and asked to indicate their preferred sequence of drug introduction in a patient with 8 weeks of symptoms. Methotrexate and low-dose prednisone were the first choice in 30% each. Hydroxychloroquine was preferred in 15%, and intra-articular steroid or another nonsteroidal anti-inflammatory drug was chosen by 10% of respondents. Gold, leflunomide, high-dose steroids, and anakinra were rarely, if ever, chosen. None of the respondents preferred a TNF-α inhibitor as the first or second choice, and combination DMARDs (with or without TNF-α inhibitors) were popular only as a tertiary choice. Despite the motto of "diagnose early and treat aggressively," these EAC rheumatologists were conservative in their approach to a patient with very early inflammatory arthritis.

Models for facilitated assessment of early rheumatoid arthritis

Fostering local or system-wide referrals of new-onset inflammatory arthritis requires forethought and effort, especially in the absence of government-supported health care systems. After listening to the growing pains and successes of several EACs in North America, the author has concluded that several key elements are needed for any early arthritis referral effort to succeed. First, there must be a commitment by the individual rheumatologist, cooperative group, or regional organization to the need and benefits of having an EAC. Second, effective promotion and education of the PCP community ensure the growth and flow of patients. The primary message must be that of facilitated access and

Table 3
Screening measures to increase the likelihood of an early inflammatory arthritis or rheumatoid arthritis diagnosis

Entry requirement	Examples	Interpretation
Minimum symptom duration	Arthritis symptoms: >6 wk >12 wk	The first few weeks of symptoms are protean. Joint symptoms for >6 wk predicts persistence, but >12 wk increases the specificity of RA.
Minimum number of swollen/tender joints	≥1 joint ≥3 joints	The likelihood of RA increases with the number of swollen joint (and persistence over time). Limited by examiners skills.
Limitations on symptom duration	<6 mo <12 mo <24 mo	Allowing patients to enter with either <6 wk or >24 mo tends to dilute the number of true RA patients. Most EACs limit symptom to either <12 mo or <6 mo. Symptoms of <6 mo may further increase the yield of RA.
Rapid access	<1 wk <2 wk <4 wk	Patients often delay seeing the physician, but when referred to the rheumatologist they are more likely to keep that appointment if the referral is immediate.
Use of physician extenders	NP PA R-RN	These can be used to screen by phone, in person, or by chart review. Referral to the rheumatologist can be driven by protocol.
PCP education	*Dear Dr* letters Newsletters Early RA conferences	First educate facilitated referral to EAC. Then educate about the urgency of early RA; education of the PCP requires ongoing efforts.
Telephone screening	5-question survey Validation of symptoms	Can be done by nonmedical personnel; ask about symptom onset, number of tender/swollen joints, family history of RA; questions to exclude OA, LBP, and fibromyalgia.
Serologic abnormalities	ESR CRP RF CCP ANA	Although may increase yield for inflammatory disease, may not be available or present in very early patients.
Prior chart review	By fax Full chart	Impediment to care; requires additional efforts by PCP/staff, rheumatologist or physician extender. May erroneously misclassify patients.
Direct referrals from colleagues	Referral form Direct telephone calls	Although single-page referral forms [2] are easy; requiring doctor-to-doctor phone contact is an impediment unless adequately promoted to colleagues.

Abbreviations: ANA, antinuclear antibody; CCP, cyclic citrullinated peptide antibody; CRP, C-reactive protein; ESR, erythrocyte sedimentation rate; LBP, low back pain; NP, nurse practitioner; OA, osteoarthritis; PA, physician assistant; R-RN, trained rheumatology nurse; RF, rheumatoid factor.

secondarily include educational exchanges on early RA and the challenge at hand. Third, a well-designed plan is needed that is achievable, reasonable, and within one's financial and manpower limitations. Lastly, all EACs should have identifiable goals. These goals may include patient recruitment for clinical studies or the earlier introduction of DMARDs or the preservation of functional or radiographic outcomes. Each of these measurable goals promotes continued buy-in by all parties—rheumatologists, PCPs, and patients.

Many rheumatologists rightfully are concerned about the return on their investment of time, resources, and finances should they consider an EAC. Establishing a facilitated early evaluation system requires expenditures and restructuring of time and resources to achieve an early and accurate diagnosis (the primary end point). Established guidelines may help ease these concerns about how to identify such patients [26,27], but algorithms that require chronicity, oligoarthritis or polyarthritis, or serologic results also may be limiting because these are often time-dependent variables. North American EACs had to learn empirically what works and what does not work. Table 3 summarizes the enrichment tools used in these EACs, with each clinic having the goal of identifying patients with early inflammatory arthritis or early RA. Several of these measures are easy to implement and would enhance the yield of early inflammatory arthritis patients, including promotional announcement letters to colleagues (*Dear Dr* letters), the use of a one-page patient referral form, requiring symptoms of greater than 6 weeks' but less than 6 months' (or 12 months') duration, cursory screens by nonmedical personnel, and guaranteeing that patients would be seen within 2 weeks of referral (see Table 3). Although many of the other commonly used tools increase the odds of having RA patients, they also conversely may impede referral of appropriate patients; this includes requiring direct physician-to-physician referrals, three or more swollen joints, screening or examinations by the rheumatologist (nurse practitioner or physician assistant), and chart reviews. The greater the need guarantee and RA referral (by employing many or restrictive tools), the fewer total referrals and fewer number of diagnosed RA patients because many with early, incomplete RA may be excluded. To optimize the "yield to effort" ratio, it may be more prudent to accept more rather than fewer referrals, using minimum but discriminatory requirements (see Table 3), to ensure that more than 10% of patients have RA or inflammatory arthritis.

Finally, not all clinicians or practice environments can absorb easily the task of remodeling their clinics to provide access to early care. Several models have been used to facilitate the initial evaluation of patients with early arthritis. Every rheumatologist has the potential to facilitate early referral; the challenge is to find the model that works best for each. Regardless of the model, the goal should be rapid consultation (ie, within 2 weeks) and a process that is easiest for the PCP to comply with. Examples include the following:

1. *Physician-to-physician request for expedited consultation:* Although most rheumatologists claim this works well for them, they fail to recognize the inherent impediments to this option (perceived delays and difficulties in

rheumatologic consultation, telephone time, PCP self-doubt), and that such measures are seldom used and hardly ever bring the very early RA patient to their attention. Nonetheless, if this is the only acceptable option for the busy practitioner, he or she should make a new or routine effort to inform colleagues of the urgency of referring such patients and setting up guidelines for what constitutes an appropriate telephone request for expedited consultation.

2. *EAC (screening) staffed by nurse practitioners or physician assistants:* In the North American EAC survey, 26% of current EACs use a physician extender, and 39% involve them voluntarily. These clinics and physician extenders operate under the guidance of a rheumatologist mentor. The physician extender responsibilities vary according to need and practice model, but may include review referral documents, screening patients by telephone, and scheduling new-onset arthritis referrals for intake, diagnostic assessments, and treatment using locally defined protocols. Research has shown efficiency, diagnostic accuracy, and patient satisfaction when nurse specialists are used as primary contacts or assessors in EACs [28–30].

3. *Dedicated EAC/time slots:* Most current dedicated EACs meet once a week and are staffed by rheumatologists and, depending on the setting, other personnel (see Table 1). Dedicated time slots for early arthritis patients can be filled weekly by scheduling staff after meeting EAC entry requirements. A half-day time commitment can allow for four or more new patients, such that more patients can be accommodated with shorter "intake screening" visits rather than a full complex evaluation. These time slots should never go unused. In the absence of an early arthritis referral, these slots may be filled from the pool of patients awaiting future consultation.

4. *Rapid EAC screens:* Some physicians prefer to facilitate referral by allowing patients to be screened rapidly with 15- to 20-minute visits when they meet entry criteria (eg, symptoms <6 months, joint pain, positive metacarpophalangeal squeeze test, or an abnormal laboratory test [CRP, ESR, RF]). These rapid screening clinics allow an astute clinician to assess supportive documents, laboratory tests, and patient intake questionnaires rapidly. The goal of these limited encounters is to answer the following questions:
   - Does the patient have inflammatory symptoms or inflammatory arthritis that merits investigation and quick follow-up?
   - Does the patient have an early autoimmune or rheumatic problem that requires rheumatologic care?
   - Does the patient have laboratory abnormalities only (eg, positive low-titer antinuclear antibody) and no rheumatic complaints that require testing or intervention?
   - Does the patient need to be referred to another provider for a non-rheumatologic condition? Rapid EAC clinics are popular with patients, who gain rapid, albeit limited, access to the specialist, and with physicians, who often can find the time to "squeeze" such patients into an existing schedule.

5. *Prescreening of early arthritis referrals:* Some practitioners allow a scheduled rapid appointment only after they have reviewed the referral sheet and supportive documents fully. This may be as simple as review of a one- page EAC referral sheet (with or without recent laboratory tests and last PCP clinic note) or as extensive as a full chart review [31] and telephone screen. In either instance, wide notice must be given of referral guidelines and process. This notice must be supplemented by PCP education and transmittal of necessary forms, documents, or records to ensure appropriate consultation.

6. *Telephone screening:* After referral by a health care provider, patients can be screened by either medical (see options 2 and 5) or by nonmedical or nursing personnel. A dedicated phone line (eg, 1-800-EARLYRA [327-5972]) and trained screener may be the most effective way of ensuring the success of regional or system-wide programs. The purpose of this model is to facilitate access, ensure transfer of necessary documents and insurance certification, verify referral symptom and symptom duration, and schedule an early visit. Nonmedical and nursing screeners can ask a limited number of questions to increase the odds of early RA and limit the number of nonurgent musculoskeletal referrals.

7. *Public relations programs:* All EAC efforts require proper notice to the intended audience (PCPs, hospital physicians, chiropractors, obstetricians, orthopedists, physical therapists) with frequent and regular reminders. Engaging PCPs in educational programs is variably effective; the use of frequent letters or newsletters may promote and educate. Consultation and involvement by a hospital public relations liaison can help develop a local or citywide strategy to promote the EAC. This promotional strategy may include local signage, features in hospital publications, newsletters, press releases, newspaper articles, media attention (radio, television, newspaper), billboards, and direct-to-consumer mailings. Although some of these publicity ideas may be costly, many are free. Promotion of EAC programs to the public always should involve the PCP as a decision maker. With education and efforts, PCP-dependent referrals are more likely to involve the patients the rheumatologist wants to see most. Even if carefully de-signed, direct-to-consumer approaches would bring scores of patients, but only a few early RA patients.

8. *Internet screening algorithms:* Several clinics have an Internet presence; however, usually these tend to be informational rather than diagnostic screening tools. Nonetheless, programs can be developed to allow patients to self-screen themselves for inflammatory arthritis, RA, or other common rheumatologic conditions. This tool allows for patient independence, use of current technology, and screening for requisite EAC or diagnostic criteria. Similar to phone screening, Internet screening should augment the odds of having RA patients (based on history and symptoms), while averting patients with less qualifying symptoms to usual methods of self-referral.

Summary

The need for rapid access to rheumatologic consultation is growing and, in certain instances, highly appropriate. There are several methods to facilitate referral and judge the risk of aggressive RA such that significant damage and disability can be averted. Practicing rheumatologists should evaluate the manner and timeline in which their rheumatoid patients currently are referred and evaluated. This article offers a variety of options and tools that can enhance efforts to promote early referral of patients with new-onset inflammatory arthritis.

Acknowledgments

The author wishes to thank the following EAC survey respondents for their input: Murray Baron (McGill Early Arthritis Registry); S. Louis Bridges (University of Alabama at Birmingham Early Arthritis Clinic); Vivian Bykerk and Edward Keystone (Toronto Early Arthritis Program); Hani El-Gabalawy (University of Manitoba); Boulos Haroui (Institut de Rhumatologie); Kevin Latinis and Bart Lindsley (Kansas University Medical Center); S. Sam Lim (Emory University/Grady Hospital); Phillip Mease (Seattle Rheumatology Associates); Steven Overman (Northwest Hospital); Stephen Paget (Hospital for Special Surgery); Janet Pope (St. Joseph's Health Care Ontario); G. Andres Quiceno and John Cush (Presbyterian Hospital of Dallas); Bernard Rubin (University of North Texas Health Science Center); H. Ralph Schumacher (University of Pennsylvania and Veterans Administration Medical Center); Carter Thorne (Southlake Regional Health Center Ontario); and David Yocum (University of Arizona). The remaining respondents chose to be anonymous.

References

[1] Emery P. Evidence supporting the benefit of early intervention in rheumatoid arthritis. J Rheumatol 2002;29(Suppl 66):3–8.
[2] Cush JJ. Early arthritis clinic: A USA perspective. Clin Exp Rheumatol 2003;21(Suppl 31): S75–8.
[3] Grigor C, Capell H, Stirling A, et al. Effect of a treatment strategy of tight control for rheumatoid arthritis (the TICORA study): a single-blind randomised controlled trial. Lancet 2004;364: 263–9.
[4] Lard LR, Visser H, Speyer I, et al. Early versus delayed treatment in patients with recent-onset rheumatoid arthritis: comparison of two cohorts who received different treatment strategies. Am J Med 2001;111:446–51.
[5] Landewe RB, Boers M, Verhoeven AC, et al. COBRA combination therapy in patients with early rheumatoid arthritis: long-term structural benefits of a brief intervention. Arthritis Rheum 2002; 46:347–56.
[6] Mottonen T, Hannonen P, Korpela M, et al. Delay to institution of therapy and induction of remission using single-drug or combination disease-modifying antirheumatic drug therapy in early rheumatoid arthritis. Arthritis Rheum 2002;46:894–8.

[7] Chan KW, Felson DT, Yood RA, Walker AM. The lag time between onset of symptoms and diagnosis of rheumatoid arthritis. Arthritis Rheum 1994;37:814–20.

[8] Irvine S, Munro R, Porter D. Early referral, diagnosis, and treatment of rheumatoid arthritis: evidence for changing medical practice. Ann Rheum Dis 1999;58:510–3.

[9] Hernandez-Garcia C, Vargas E, Abasolo L, et al. Lag time between onset of symptoms and access to rheumatology care and DMARD therapy in a cohort of patients with rheumatoid arthritis. J Rheumatol 2000;27:2323–8.

[10] Soderlin MK, Borjesson O, Kautiainen H, et al. Annual incidence of inflammatory joint diseases in a population based study in southern Sweden. Ann Rheum Dis 2002;61:911–5.

[11] Wiles N, Symmons DP, Harrison B, et al. Estimating the incidence of rheumatoid arthritis: trying to hit a moving target? Arthritis Rheum 1999;42:1339–46.

[12] Doran MF, Pond GR, Crowson CS, et al. Trends in incidence and mortality in rheumatoid arthritis in Rochester, Minnesota, over a forty-year period. Arthritis Rheum 2002;46:625–31.

[13] Nell VP, Machold KP, Eberl G, et al. Benefit of very early referral and very early therapy with disease-modifying anti-rheumatic drugs in patients with early rheumatoid arthritis. Rheumatology (Oxf) 2004;43:906–14.

[14] Egsmose C, Lund B, Borg G, et al. Patients with rheumatoid arthritis benefit from early 2nd line therapy: 5-year follow up of a prospective double blind placebo controlled study. J Rheumatol 1995;22:2208–13.

[15] Pincus T, Gibofsky A, Weinblatt ME. Urgent care and tight control of rheumatoid arthritis as in diabetes and hypertension: better treatments but a shortage of rheumatologists. Arthritis Rheum 2002;46:851–4.

[16] Hallert E, Husberg M, Jonsson D, Skogh T. Rheumatoid arthritis is already expensive during the first year of the disease (the Swedish TIRA project). Rheumatology (Oxf) 2004;43:1374–82.

[17] Puolakka K, Kautiainen H, Mottonen T, et al. FIN-RACo trial group: predictors of productivity loss in early rheumatoid arthritis: a 5 year follow up study. Ann Rheum Dis 2005;64:130–3.

[18] Jansen LM, van der Horst-Bruinsma I, Lems WF, et al. Serological bone markers and joint damage in early polyarthritis. J Rheumatol 2004;31:1491–6.

[19] Rantapaa-Dahlqvist S, de Jong BA, Berglin E, et al. Antibodies against cyclic citrullinated peptide and IgA rheumatoid factor predict the development of rheumatoid arthritis. Arthritis Rheum 2003;48:2741–9.

[20] Fuchs HA, Kaye JJ, Callahan LF, et al. Evidence of significant radiographic damage in rheumatoid arthritis within the first 2 years of disease. J Rheumatol 1989;16:585–91.

[21] Sokka T, Willoughby J, Yazici Y, Pincus T. Databases of patients with early rheumatoid arthritis in the USA. Clin Exp Rheumatol 2003;21(Suppl 31):S146–53.

[22] Bathon JM, Martin RW, Fleischmann RM, et al. A comparison of etanercept and methotrexate in patients with early rheumatoid arthritis. N Engl J Med 2000;343:1586–93.

[23] St. Clair EW, van der Heijde D, Smolen J, et al. Combination infliximab and methotrexate therapy for early rheumatoid arthritis: a randomized controlled trial. Arthritis Rheum 2004;50: 3432–43.

[24] Breedveld FC, Kavanaugh AF, Cohen SB, et al. Early treatment of rheumatoid arthritis (RA) with adalimumab (HUMIRA) plus methotrexate vs. adalimumab alone or methotrexate alone: the PREMIER study. Arthritis Rheum 2004;50(Suppl):L5.

[25] Cush JJ. Cytokine inhibitors. In: Hochberg MC, Silman AJ, Smolen JS, et al, editors. Rheumatology. 3rd edition. Edinburgh: Mosby; 2003. p. 461–84.

[26] Cush JJ. Early arthritis clinics: if you build it will they come? J Rheumatol 2005;32:203–7.

[27] Emery P, Breedveld FC, Dougados M, et al. Early referral recommendation for newly diagnosed rheumatoid arthritis: evidence based development of a clinical guide. Ann Rheum Dis 2002;61: 290–7.

[28] Gradwell C, Thomas KS, English JS, Williams HC. A randomized controlled trial of nurse follow-up clinics: do they help patients and do they free up consultants' time? Br J Dermatol 2002;147:513–7.

[29] Tijhuis GJ, Zwinderman AH, Hazes JM, et al. A randomized comparison of care provided by a

clinical nurse specialist, an inpatient team, and a day patient team in rheumatoid arthritis. Arthritis Rheum 2002;47:525–31.

[30] Gormley GJ, Steele WK, Gilliland A, et al. Can diagnostic triage by general practitioners or rheumatology nurses improve the positive predictive value of referrals to early arthritis clinics? Rheumatology (Oxf) 2003;42:763–8.

[31] Newman ED, Harrington TM, Olenginski TP, et al. "The rheumatologist can see you now": successful implementation of an advanced access model in a rheumatology practice. Arthritis Rheum 2004;51:253–7.

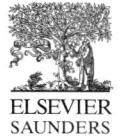

ELSEVIER
SAUNDERS

RHEUMATIC
DISEASE CLINICS
OF NORTH AMERICA

Rheum Dis Clin N Am 31 (2005) 605–626

Early Undifferentiated Arthritis

Carol A. Hitchon, MD, FRCPC, MSc,
Christine A. Peschken, MD, FRCPC, MSc,
Saeed Shaikh, MD, FRCPC,
Hani S. El-Gabalawy, MD, FRCPC*

Department of Medicine, University of Manitoba and Arthritis Center, Winnipeg, MB, Canada

Population-based cohorts of early inflammatory arthritis from the 1950s and 1960s identified a group of patients with seronegative benign polyarthritis who had complete or near-complete resolution of symptoms after several years [1]. More recently, with the establishment of early arthritis clinics, it has become clear that a sizable proportion of patients with early inflammatory arthritis cannot be classified into a specific diagnosis using the traditional American College of Rheumatology (ACR) criteria [2]. The outcome of these patients varies. The term "undifferentiated arthritis" (UA) subsequently was proposed to emphasize the heterogeneity of these unclassifiable arthritides and their potential to evolve into a definable form of arthritis. Zeidler et al [3] categorized undifferentiated arthritis further into several subgroups based on clinical outcome. A patient with UA may have an early stage of a defined arthritis that will meet criteria in time, a forme fruste or partial form of a classifiable disease, an overlap of more than one disease entity, or an arthritis of unknown origin that may (or may not) become differentiated in the future. The heterogeneity associated with the term "UA" emphasizes the need for continued follow-up and reassessment of the diagnosis and management of these patients. Clinicians need tools to predict outcome in this group to initiate appropriate therapy. These tools can be developed through

* Corresponding author. Department of Medicine, University of Manitoba, Arthritis Center, RR149 800 Sherbrook Street, Winnipeg, MB R3A 1M4, Canada.

E-mail address: elgabal@cc.umanitoba.ca (H.S. El-Gabalawy).

0889-857X/05/$ – see front matter © 2005 Elsevier Inc. All rights reserved.
doi:10.1016/j.rdc.2005.07.006
rheumatic.theclinics.com

an increased understanding of the pathologic events contributing to persistent synovitis and through clinical studies of early arthritis cohorts.

Prevalence of undifferentiated arthritis

The prevalence of UA can be estimated from cohorts of early inflammatory arthritis; however, these estimates vary depending on the disease duration at the time of assessment and the inclusion criteria of each cohort. Inception cohorts from Europe and North America have shown that UA is common and seen more frequently than rheumatoid arthritis (RA) (Table 1). Estimates range from 7% to 60% of early arthritis cohorts. This proportion decreases with increasing disease duration probably because a proportion of UA patients ultimately develop classifiable arthritis, such as RA, spondyloarthropathy, psoriatic arthritis, or reactive arthritis. Disease prevalence based on clinic populations likely underestimates true population prevalence because even in health care systems with highly integrated early arthritis clinics and self-referral programs, a proportion of the population is not evaluated.

Few studies have reported incidence rates for UA. In their study of RA incidence, Wiles et al [4] found that RA incidence increases (and UA incidence decreases) with increasing disease duration. In Sweden, an annual incidence rate for all inflammatory arthritis (mean symptom duration 2 months; range 0–17 months) was 115 per 100,000. Of these, the incidence rate for UA was 54 per 100,000 compared with 31 per 100,000 for RA, 28 per 100,000 for reactive arthritis, and less than 10 per 100,000 for other arthropathies [5] An annual incidence rate for all adult inflammatory arthritis in Finland was 271 per 100,000 with incidence rates for UA and RA of 148.5 per 100,000 and 36.1 per 100,000 [6]. The difference between these two studies may be due to the inclusion of children in the Finland study. In the Nurses Health Study ($n = 116,779$ American women), 344 new cases of polyarthritis were identified (RA 98.5/100,000, UA 87.3/100,000, non-RA 108.8/100,000) [7]. Clinicians potentially see at least as much if not more recent-onset UA than recent-onset RA.

Clinical presentation of undifferentiated arthritis

UA often presents more acutely than RA [8]. The total affected joint count (particularly swollen joint count) is usually lower with less hand involvement and less symmetric joint involvement. Oligoarthritis, particularly of large joints, is common, occurring in half of patients at presentation and after extended follow-up (see later). In addition, the duration of early morning stiffness is often shorter, and functional disability as measured by the Health Assessment Questionnaire or grip strength is sometimes significantly less [9,10] Despite these differences in joint involvement, patient measures of the degree of pain and disease activity are often similar to the measures reported in early RA. The acute phase response measured by erythrocyte sedimentation rate (ESR) or C-reactive protein (CRP) may be similar or lower than in RA with the exception of serum amyloid A levels, which are higher in RA [11].

A proportion of early UA patients, particularly patients with acute oligo-arthritis, may represent reactive arthritis despite not having a clear history of preceding infection. In these cases, a thorough search for offending organisms may be beneficial. In a cohort of early arthritis patients with less than 3 months of symptoms, a preceding infection with any of a wide variety of organisms was found in 45% of patients and was associated with an increased chance of remission after 6 months, suggesting a diagnosis of reactive arthritis [12] Other investigators have found evidence of preceding bacterial exposure through culture, serology [13,14], or DNA testing [15] in 30% to 50% of early undifferentiated oligoarthritis. Infection should be sought out by history and physical examination. Appropriate cultures and serology should be obtained because cultures, particularly for infections such as *Chlamydia,* may be more sensitive than serologic testing [13]. When a thorough search for infection has been completed and found negative, however, individuals should be classified as having UA and not reactive arthritis and risk stratified for disease severity.

Role of imaging in the assessment of undifferentiated arthritis

Radiographic evidence of joint erosions and joint space narrowing are late findings that generally represent irreversible damage. Such changes are more common in early RA than early UA [16,17], but can be seen in 35% of poly-articular UA (possibly less for oligoarticular UA) at presentation [18–20]. Studies suggest that erosions can develop in one third of patients, although estimates range from less than 5% to 77% depending on the population characteristics and duration of follow-up [17,21]. Radiographic erosions present within the first year of disease are strong predictors of future damage.

Sensitive imaging modalities such as ultrasound and MRI that can detect and quantify synovitis, vascularity, and bone marrow changes preceding radiographic bone erosions currently are being developed and evaluated in early arthritis [22,23]. MRI is much more sensitive than radiography for detecting bone erosions and is able to detect synovitis and bone marrow edema, which precede bone erosions. Ultrasound is able to detect synovitis better than clinical examination, and with the use of power Doppler, synovial vascularity can be assessed. Issues related to methodology and standardized guidelines for interpretation are still in development for both techniques. Given the flexibility to examine multiple joints at a time in the clinic and potentially greater accessibility, ultrasound is likely to be a more logistically viable imaging modality for evaluating and monitoring treatment response than MRI.

Table 1
Prevalence and prognosis of undifferentiated arthritis in selected cohort studies

First author, year [Ref.]; (location/cohort name)	Study size[a]	Symptom duration at enrollment	Follow-up	Outcome of UA
Machold, 2002 [8]; (Vienna, Austria)	Total = 108 RA = 61% UA = 28%	≤3 mo	1 y	Resolved = 61% RA = 27% Other disease = 3% Persistent UA = 19%
Woolf, 1991 [68] and Hall, 1982 [69]; (Bath, UK)[b]	Total = 88 Polyarthritis = 55% Oligoarthritis = 45% *Initial 76 recruited:* RA = 33 or 43% UA = 43 or 57%	<3 mo	Minimum 5 y	Remission = 30% Persistent = 70% Final diagnosis: RA = 36 or 41% UA = 6 or 7% Remission = 3 or 50% Persistent UA = 50% Other = 51%
Raza, 2005 [62]; (Birmingham, UK)	Total = 96 RA = 24 or 25% UA = 72 or 75%	<3 mo	18 mo	Remission = 45% Persistent UA = 19% Other disease = 35%
Tunn, 1993 [61]; Salmon, 1993 [40]; and Gough, 1994 [38]; (Birmingham, UK)	Total = 65 UA = 58%	<6 mo	4 y	At 1 y: Resolved = 55% At 4 y: Resolved: 27% RA = 49% Persistent UA = 24%
Ioaoui, 2004 [53]; (France)	Monoarthritis = 46 UA = 16 or 35% Probable diagnosis = 30 or 65%	Mean 10 mo	6 y	Remission = 10 or 63% Specific arthropathy = 5 or 31% Persistent UA = 1 or 6%

Study	Inclusion (duration)	Follow-up	Outcome
Kvein, 1996 [44]; (Oslo, Norway) Oligoarthritis=146 *Diagnosis at 24 wk:* ReA=46 or 32% UA=62 or 42% Noninflammatory=15 or 10% Other inflammatory=17 or 15%	<2 mo	24 wk	Remission ≈90% Persistent UA (swelling) ≈10%
Wolfe, 1993 [10]; (Wichita, KS) Total=1141 RA=503 or 44% UA=638 or 56%	≤2 y ≤6 mo	>3 y	Resolved=20% RA=15% Other disease=20% Persistent UA=10%
Nissila, 1983 [63] and Kaarala, 1985 [64]; (Heinola, Finland) Total=376 RA=107 or 28% UA=161 or 43% AS/ReA=84 or 22% PsA=14 or 4% CTD=10 or 3%	<6 mo	3 y	ND
Zeidler, 1995 [3]; (Germany) Total=217 RA=41 or 19% UA=117 or 54% SpA=11 or 5%	<1 y	4–38 mo	Resolved=24% RA=7% Persistent UA=36%
Harrison, 2000 [51] and 1996 [70]; (Norfolk Arthritis Registry cohort) Total=532 (354 with 2-y follow-up in 1996) RA=254 or 72% UA=100 or 28%	<1 y	2 y	Of 100 UA: Resolved=19 or 19% Persistent=58 or 58% Remission=23 or 23%

(continued on next page)

Table 1 (*continued*)

First author, year [Ref.]; (location/cohort name)	Study size[a]	Symptom duration at enrollment	Follow-up	Outcome of UA
Glennas, 2000 [9]; (Oslo, Norway)	Total=92 RA=48% UA=41% of which 11% oligoarthritis/PMR UA=100 or 28%	<26 y	5 y	ND Persistent=58 or 58% Remission=23 or 23%
Vittecoq, 2004 [34]; (France)	Total=314 RA=179 or 57% UA=75 or 24% Other=63 or 20%	<6 mo	—	ND
Morel, 2000 [71]; (Montpellier, France)	Total=43 UA=all or 100%	<1 y	>1 y	RA=42% Remission=28%
Quinn, 2003 [59] and Green, 1999 and 2001 [43,58]; (Leeds, UK)	Total=1877 (56% with inflammatory arthritis) RA=526 or 50% UA=242 or 23% (97 followed) SPA/PsA=137 or 13% Other=147 or 14%	<1 y	1 y	*Follow up on 97 UA patients (with hand involvement):* Remission: 13 or 13% RA=14 or 14% Other=38 or 39% Persistent synovitis=35 or 36%
El-Gabalawy, 1999 [18] and Goldbach-Mansky, 2000 [24]; (National Institutes of Health cohort)	Total=211 UA=75 or 36% RA=98 or 46% SPA=38 or 18%	<1 y	1 y	ND

Reference			
Mau, 1989 [72]	Total=141 RA=57 or 40% UA=40 or 28% SPA/other=44 or 31%	<1 y	—	UA/SPA persistent disease=32% Remission=68% (did not separate SPA from UA)
Schumacher, 2004 [56]; (Pennsylvania, PA)	Total=121 *Diagnosis at 1 y:* RA=20 or 17% UA=59 or 49% SpA=18 or 15% Other=24 or 20%	<1 y	>1 y (median 5 y)	Remission=40 or 67% Persistent UA=19 or 32%
Higami, 1997 [21]; (Tokyo, Japan)	Total=198 RA=82 or 41% UA=116 or 59%	<1 y	1 y	UA reexamined=96 RA=40 or 42%
Jacobsen, 2001 [73]; Jensen, 2004 [19]; and Klarlund, 2000 [17] (TIRA Group/Denmark)	Total=72 RA=44% UA (polyarthritis)=28%	<2 y	2 y	RA=28%
van Gaalen, 2004 [20]; (Leidin, The Netherlands)	Total=936 RA=205 or 22% UA=346 or 37% Other=385 or 41%	<2 y	3 y	RA=40%
Vos, 2001 [41]; (Leidin, The Netherlands)	Total=548 *Diagnosis at 1 y:* RA=158 or 29% UA=138 or 25% Other=207 or 38%	—	2 y	Remission=70%

(continued on next page)

Table 1 (*continued*)

First author, year [Ref.]; (location/cohort name)	Study size[a]	Symptom duration at enrollment	Follow-up	Outcome of UA
Jansen, 2002 [60]; (Amsterdam, The Netherlands)	Total = 280 UA = 77 or 27% RA = 203 or 72%	<3 y	1 y	Progressive UA = 27% Mild UA = 58% RA = 13% Resolved = % not stated
Jansen, 2002 [25] and Nielen, 2005 [74]; (Amsterdam, The Netherlands)	Total = 379 *Diagnosis at 1 y:* RA = 258 or 68% UA = 121 or 32%	Mean 4.8 mo	—	Polyarthritis = 60% Oligoarthritis = 40%

Abbreviations: ND; not done; TIRA, (in Danish) early rheumatoid arthritis.
  [a] Where several publications report on the same cohort, largest cohort size recorded.
  [b] Follow-up for whole cohort (not specific for UA).

Role of rheumatoid arthritis–associated antibodies in the assessment of undifferentiated arthritis

UA patients are less likely to have elevated levels of RA-specific autoantibodies than RA patients. IgM rheumatoid factor is positive in 6% to 20% of UA patients; IgA rheumatoid factor is positive in 6%, and cyclic citrullinated peptide (CCP) is positive in 3% to 20% [20,24,25]. The presence of rheumatoid factor (RF), in particular IgA RF, seems to be associated with more severe disease, and IgM RF can predict erosions, persistent disease, and future RA with variable accuracy in early arthritis cohorts.

The presence of RA-specific antibodies of potential pathologic significance to inflammatory arthritis, in particular CCP, has been incorporated into several models to predict outcome in early arthritis (although not specific for early UA) [26–29]. In most of these models, CCP, in combination with various other clinical variables, predicted disease persistence, progression, or development of erosions and in some studies disability after follow-up of 5 years, often with greater accuracy than RF, although the clinical usefulness of CCP may be most beneficial in RF-negative patients [30]. One model to predict persistent erosive disease in an individual patient has been described using the Leiden early arthritis cohort with initial confirmation in the Norfolk Arthritis Registry (NOAR) cohort. Included variables (symptom duration, morning stiffness, arthritis in three joint groups, metatarsophalangeal compression pain, IgM RF, and CCP) are scored and summed to provide an estimate of predictive value with reasonable discriminating ability (area under the receiver operating curve 0.83) [29,31]. In an expanded Leiden cohort of 936 patients, 127 of 318 UA patients progressed to RA. In these UA patients, CCP and ACR criteria, specifically polyarthritis, symmetric arthritis, and erosions, predicted the development of RA [20]. These studies indicate that in early UA, CCP, in combination with clinical variables, identifies patients requiring closer follow-up and potentially more aggressive therapy.

Additional RA-specific autoantibodies have been studied, including anti-Sa, which targets citrullinated vimentin [32] and seems to identify patients with greater potential for erosive disease [33], and anticitrullinated rat filaggrin, which is specific for early RA [34]. The clinical utility of these and other antibodies to citrullinated peptides remains to be determined [24].

Inflammation and oxidative stress cause protein damage through nonenzymatic glycosylation pathways, leading to the formation of advanced glycosylation end products (AGE). In diabetes, hemoglobin AGE is a clinically useful predictor of vascular complications. AGE products have been shown in established RA, and levels have correlated with various measures of disease activity. AGE-damaged IgG (AGE-IgG) and antibodies to AGE-IgG (anti–AGE-IgG) were studied in the National Institutes of Health (NIH) early arthritis cohort [35]. AGE-IgG was present in 20% of patients regardless of diagnosis and associated with greater disease activity (ESR, CRP). RA patients, particularly patients with RF, were more likely to have persistently elevated anti–AGE-IgG titers, however, than UA patients, who had only transiently elevated anti–AGE-IgG levels. The role of anti–AGE-IgG in prognosis needs further evaluation.

Role of HLA testing in the assessment of undifferentiated arthritis

The shared epitope doubles the risk of developing RA in population studies, an association that is even stronger in individuals with antibodies to citrullinated peptides [36], and is associated with erosions and RF [18,37]. Up to 32% of UA patients have the shared epitope, a similar frequency as seen in RF-negative RA, and HLA-DQβ1 0302 may be underrepresented in early UA compared with other arthropathies [18]. Studies in early cohorts including UA patients have shown variable associations (or lack thereof) between the HLA-DRβ1 shared epitope and disease persistence or severity of erosions [21,38–40]. It has been proposed that the HLA-DRβ1 shared epitope and the HLA-DQβ1 molecules DQ3 and DQ5 increase susceptibility to RA, whereas in patients with DQ5, the presence HLA-DRβ1 molecules with a specific peptide sequence (DERAA) in their hypervariable region may protect against severe RA [37,41]. UA is associated with the potentially protective DQ5, but not DQ3, and UA patients were more likely to have DQ3 with the protective DERAA than DQ3 alone [42]. The shared epitope also has been associated with early treatment response in one cohort [43]. These data suggest that HLA typing including the shared epitope, DQ3, DQ5, and DERAA may be beneficial in early disease if these initial reports are confirmed in other cohorts.

HLA-B27 is present in 16% of early UA patients and in 29% of patients meeting European Spondyloarthropathy Study Group (ESSG) criteria for spondyloarthropathy [18]. UA patients presenting with oligoarthritis who are B27 positive in combination with CRP, genitourinary symptoms, and metatarsal pain are more likely to develop reactive arthritis [44].

Role of synovial biopsy in the assessment of undifferentiated arthritis

Synovial tissue can be obtained by closed needle biopsy or by arthroscopy. Both techniques are invasive and time-consuming to perform requiring variable amounts of technical expertise, limiting widespread clinical use. Despite these limitations, arthroscopy and biopsy are valuable tools to assess pathologic events in arthritis.

The tortuous blood vessels described at the time of arthroscopy in early psoriatic arthritis and spondyloarthropathy differ from the relatively straight vessels of RA [45] and seem to be preserved over time regardless of treatment [46]. Early UA patients were more likely to have tortuous or a mixed pattern of vessels (76%). Six UA patients developed a specific arthropathy (four RA and two who had a straight pattern, 1 psoriatic arthritis and 1 spondyloarthropathy, both with tortuous patterns). In this study, the straight vascular pattern had a sensitivity of 77% and specificity of 70% for RA.

Synovial tissue analysis provides insight into the pathologic events contributing to disease progression and may be beneficial in predicting diagnosis and prognosis [47,48]. In early arthritis, histologic evidence of increased numbers of B cells and plasma cells and integrin expression was able to differentiate RA from non-RA, although none of these features were specific enough to assign diagnosis and were unlikely to be clinically useful. The presence of CCP in synovium, which has greater direct relevance to underlying disease pathogenesis, is much more specific for RA and likely to be of greater benefit in distinguishing RA from other arthropathies in early undifferentiated disease [49].

Synovial biopsy features also can be used to assess prognosis [48]. Studies in early RA showed that radiographic erosions were associated with increased macrophage numbers and matrix metalloproteinases. In the NIH cohort including UA and RA patients, persistent synovitis at 1 year was predicted by the presence of several histopathologic features, including the presence of stromal fibrin deposition, stromal mesenchymal transformation, microvascular damage, lymphoid organization with lymphoid follicles and high endothelial blood vessels, and tissue necrosis. The presence of high endothelial blood vessels, lymphoid follicles, and microvascular damage were highly associated with RA-specific autoantibodies [50]. In addition to assisting with prognosis, these pathologic associations provide clues to the mechanisms associated with persistent disease.

Determining prognosis of early undifferentiated arthritis

The key question facing clinicians seeing patients with UA relates to determining prognosis. In particular, whether the patient's synovitis will remit, persist, result in erosive joint damage with functional impairment, or, perhaps less importantly, whether criteria for RA or another defined arthritis will be met in the future. Studies of outcome must be interpreted after the duration of symptoms at enrollment, the clinical characteristics of patients enrolled, and the duration of follow-up are considered because these variables all influence findings.

Many studies have investigated the outcome of early arthritis; however, most have included only RA patients or have not reported outcomes specific to UA, and differences in study population limit widespread applicability of the results [31,51,52]. These studies provide some indication of prognosis and predictors of prognosis applicable to early arthritis in general if not specific for UA. Estimates of prognosis from studies specifically reporting outcomes for UA suggest that 13% to 60% of UA patients experience remission, 7% to 65% evolve into RA or another definable disease, and 10% to 40% have persistent disease activity, but remain undifferentiated (see Table 1). A review has shown that monarthritis, in particular, goes into remission in 60% of cases, progresses to chronic oligoarthritis or polyarthritis in 10% to 40% of cases, and remains undifferentiated in 70% of cases [53].

Table 2
Predictors of prognosis in cohorts of undifferentiated arthritis using multivariate analysis

First author, year [Ref.]; (location/cohort name)	Sample size	Erosion	Persistence	Rheumatoid arthritis
Wolfe, 1993 [10]; (KS)	Total = 1141 RA = 44 UA = 56%	ND	RF, symptom duration at first visit, ACR criteria	ND
Nielen, 2005 [74]; (Amsterdam, The Netherlands)	Total = 379 RA = 258 UA = 121	Accuracy=80% CCP baseline erosion, ESR	ND	CCP, RF, ACF, DAS pain Accuracy=78%
Van Gaalen [20][a]; (Leiden, UK)	Total = 936 UA = 318 (future RA = 127) RA = 205	ND	ND	ACR criteria CCP, CCP most benefit with more ACR criteria AUC = 0.92
Vittecoq, 2004 [34]; (Very Early Inflammatory Arthritis cohort)	ND	ND	ND	ACRF predicts RA better than RF and CCP
Fardellone, 2003 [75] and Vittecoq, 2003 [76,77][b]; (Very Early Inflammatory Arthritis cohort)	Total ≈ 314 Diagnosis at 1 y: RA = 176 UA = 75 Other = 63	Accuracy = 79% IgG RF, baseline erosion, pain AUC = 0.74	IgM RF, Ritchie index (varied with definition of remission)	CCP, SJC, grip strength, APN AUC = 0.84
Green, 1999 and 2001 [43,58] and Quinn, 2003 [59]; (Leeds, UK)	Total = 63 Diagnosis at 6 mo: RA = 32 or 65% UA = 10 or 20% Other inflammatory = 10%	ND	6 mo: duration <12 wk (OR 4.9)	ND

Study	Population			Predictors
Harrison, 2000 [51]; (Norfolk Arthritis Registry)	Total = 486 RA = 231 or 48% Other IP = 255 or 52%	RF duration >3 mo Accuracy = 70% PPV = 60% NPV = 76%	RF, polyarthritis ankle swelling Accuracy = 74% PPV = 63% NPV = 80%	ND
Jansen, 2002 [60][a]; (Amsterdam, The Netherlands)	Total = 280 UA = 77 or 27% RA = 208 or 72%	ND	Age[a] (OR 1.05) Hand arthritis (OR 4.2)	No significant predictors[a]
Kvien, 1996 [44]; (Oslo, Norway)	Total = 146 ReA = 46 UA = 62 Other = 38 RA = excluded	ND	ND	ReA, HLAB27, MTP genitourinary symptoms, CRP
Raza, 2005 [62]; (Birmingham, UK)	Total = 96 UA = 47 RA = 24 Other = 25	ND	ND	RF, CCP, age, polyarthritis
Tunn, 1993 [61]; (Birmingham, UK)	Toal = 65 Diagnosis not given	ND	RF, ESR Sensitivity = 69% Specificity = 94%	ND

Abbreviations: ACRF, anticitrullinated rat filaggrin; APN, antiperinuclear factor; AUC, area under the receiver operating curve; MTP, metatarsophalangeal; ND, not done; NVP, negative predictive value; PPV, positive predictive value; ReA, reactive arthritis, SIC, swollen joint count.

[a] Specifically looked at prognosis of UA.

[b] Published in abstract form only.

Studies of undifferentiated arthritis outcome from cohorts around the world

Cohort studies of early inflammatory arthritis, including RA and UA, have identified multiple clinical features and laboratory investigations associated with disease persistence, the development of erosions, functional status, or a final diagnosis of RA or other arthropathy (Table 2). Many individual clinical features, although suggestive, are not sufficiently reliable to predict disease persistence accurately in an individual patient, and the predictive value of many clinical features has not been confirmed in multivariate models. Of the variables that have been evaluated with multivariate models, the presence of RA autoantibodies, in particular RF and CCP [54,55]; baseline functional status; shared epitope; polyarthritis with hand or foot involvement [29,56]; duration of symptoms at presentation; and erosions at presentation seem to be the strongest predictors of disease persistence, progression of erosions, development into RA or another definable arthropathy or future disability [31,51,52]. Some of the clinical features shown to be predictive of disease persistence form part of the criteria used to make a diagnosis of RA or spondyloarthropathy, supporting the suggestion that some cases of UA are incomplete forms of another diagnostic disease. Progression from UA to RA has been shown to be more likely in patients with subacute symptoms, polyarthritis, the presence of RF and shared epitope, and resistance to initial corticosteroid (or contemporary disease-modifying antirheumatic drug [DMARD]) treatment. The presence of antibodies to CCP has been found to be an even better predictor of future RA than RF [57]. Similarly, progression from undifferentiated oligoarthritis to reactive arthritis was predicted by the combination of CRP, genitourinary symptoms, metatarsal pain, and HLA-B27 with a sensitivity of 69% and a specificity of 94% [44]. Few cohorts have evaluated prognostic features in early UA separate from RA.

In the Leeds early arthritis cohort, patients are treated using a structured management protocol. Disease duration of greater than 12 weeks was the strongest predictor of persistent disease at 6 months (for RA and UA) [43]. In a separate analysis of early oligoarthritis, failure to respond to corticosteroids within 2 weeks predicted persistent disease at 12 weeks (occurring in 55%), whereas persistent disease at 1 year (occurring in 49%) was predicted by the 2-week treatment response, RF, and a longer disease duration [58]. In patients with early, undifferentiated polyarthritis of the hands, the presence of synovitis at 12 weeks predicted the need for DMARDs (required by 30%) over the course of 1 year. RF and the painful joint count predicted progression to RA [59]. CCP was not evaluated.

Jansen et al [60] in Amsterdam evaluated the outcome of 280 patients with early (<3 years) inflammatory arthritis (RA 72%, UA 27%). After 1 year, 42% of UA patients had progressive disease predicted by increasing age and hand involvement. Patients with mild UA had lower disease activity scores at onset, but this was not found to be significant in multivariate analysis. RA developed in 16% of UA patients, and although these patients had less RF, lower CRP, and less disease activity than progressive UA, not meeting criteria for RA, no predictors were identified on multivariate analysis. The predictive role of CCP antibodies was not evaluated in this study; however, in a larger cohort from the same center (379 patients; RA 68%, UA 32%), CCP and IgM RF predicted RA at presentation with a sensitivity of 55% and a specificity of 97% [25], and baseline CCP predicted the development of erosions (combined UA and RA) [26].

Predictors of persistent synovitis in a cohort of patients with early polyarthritis ($n = 65$; RA 49%, non-RA 51%) were examined in two reports from Birmingham. RF and ESR best predicted persistent disease (in RA and non-RA) after 1 year, whereas the presence of shared epitope DR4 or DR1 (or both) was seen more commonly in patients who progressed to persistent RA at 4 years [40,61]. In a subsequent cohort (< 3 months; UA 75%, RA 25%) from the same group, age, symmetric arthritis, RF, and CCP predicted the development of persistent RA from a cohort of UA and RA [62].

Schumacher's [56] Pennsylvania cohort of 121 early arthritis patients (mean disease duration of 3 months; monarthritis 21%, oligoarthritis 34%, polyarthritis 45%) were followed for at least 1 year (median 5 years). Of patients, 52% were in remission (a third who had a transient synovitis of < 6 months' duration), and 45% had persistently active disease. Although the clinical diagnosis at presentation was not provided, according to the final diagnosis, 50% of UA patients had persistent disease compared with 90% of RA and 85% of spondyloarthropathy patients. Polyarthritis with hand involvement best predicted persistent disease in a combined analysis of RA and UA; however, laboratory investigations, including acute-phase response, evidence of preceding infection, and RF status, did not predict remission with any reliability in an individual patient.

Wolfe's [10] study from Kansas included patients with polyarthritis of less than 2 years' duration ($n = 1141$; RA 44%, UA 56%) and found that UA patients had shorter symptom duration at presentation, less RF, lower ESR, fewer nodules, less joint swelling, and less functional disability than RA patients. On follow-up, more than half of the UA patients (54%) experienced resolution by 18 months, and 17% developed RA. Patients with RF, increasing duration of symptoms at presentation, and ACR criteria for RA were less likely to experience resolution and more likely to develop RA.

Nissila and Kaarela [63,64] reported outcomes from the Heinola cohort of early arthritis established in 1973. After 3 years, UA patients had less joint involvement, fewer erosions, and better functional ability and were more likely to be working than RA patients. HLA-B27 patients had the best prognosis. Specific predictors of outcome were reported after 8 years of follow-up, and the number of joints involved at onset was one of the best predictors of outcome.

Kvien et al [44] reported predictors of a diagnosis of reactive arthritis in a cohort of initially undifferentiated oligoarthritis. In this study, one of the few to report specifically on reactive arthritis as a final diagnosis, reactive arthritis developed in 32%, and 42% remained undifferentiated. Reactive arthritis and UA had a good course with most patients (> 80%) experiencing resolution of arthritis and acute-phase response by 24 weeks.

The authors have evaluated the course of patients with persistent undifferentiated disease by comparing the clinical features of patients with recent-onset

Table 3

Clinical characteristics of oligoarticular and polyarticular undifferentiated arthritis of at least 3 years duration

Clinical characteristics	Oligoarticular ($n = 42$)	Polyarticular ($n = 44$)	P value
Age (y)	43	49	<0.001
Female (%)[a]	57	84	0.006
Affected joint count[b]	1.67	16.11	<0.001
DMARD (%)[a]	30	66	<0.001
Prednisone (%)[a]	5	15	NS
Sacroilititis (%)[a]	23	7	0.03
mHAQ[b]	0.47	0.71	0.07

Mean = 11 y.

Abbreviations: mHAQ, modified Health Assessment Questionnaire; NS, not significant.

[a] Chi squared.
[b] Mann Whitney U.

early UA of less than 1 year's duration (NIH inception cohort, $n = 75$; University of Manitoba cohort, $n = 71$; total $n = 146$) with a cohort of patients with persistent UA of more than 3 years' duration (University of Manitoba cohort, $n = 86$). Spondyloarthropathies specifically were excluded. In this combined cohort of early UA patients, most had oligoarthritis, more than a third were taking DMARDs, and 7% had erosions. The features of the long-standing UA cohort were compared with the cohort of early UA and are shown in Table 3. The mean follow-up of patients with persistent UA was 11 years. Nearly half had oligoarthritis, and nearly a third had monarthritis. The most commonly affected joints in patients with persistent oligoarthritis were the knees, and the most commonly affected joints in patients with persistent polyarthritis were the wrists. Compared with patients with persistent oligoarthritis, patients with persistent undifferentiated polyarthritis were more likely to be female, to have symmetric joint involvement, to have poorer functional status, and to be taking DMARDs, whereas patients with persistent oligoarthritis were more likely to have sacroiliitis. Compared with early UA patients, persistent UA patients were older, had more involved joints, and had greater disability (Table 4).

Table 4

Comparison of early and longstanding undifferentiated arthritis

Clinical characteristics	Early UA ($n = 146$)	Late UA ($n = 86$)	P value
Age (y)[a]	40	46	<0.001
Female (%)[b]	65	71	NS
Affected joint count[a]	2.3	8.9	<0.001
Oligoarthritis (%)[b]	71	49	<0.002
DMARD use (%)	37	47	NS
mHAQ[a]	0.31	0.59	0.001

Abbreviations: mHAQ, modified Health Assessment Questionnaire; NS, not significant.

[a] Mann Whitney U.
[b] Chi squared.

Table 5
Comparison of late undifferentiated arthritis with rheumatoid arthritis of similar disease duration

Clinical characteristics	Late UA ($n = 86$)	Late RA ($n = 621$)	P value
Age (y)[a]	46	57	<0.001
Disease duration (y)[a]	11	12	NS
Affected jointsa	9	30	<0.001
RF+ (%)[b]	14	96	<0.001
DMARD (%)[b]	47	99	<0.001
Prednisone(%)[b]	11	29	<0.001
mHAQ[a]	0.59	0.82	0.003
Self-reported employment (% full-time UA)[a]	36	16	<0.001

Abbreviations: mHAQ, modified Health Assessment Questionnaire; NS, not significant; RF+, rheumatoid-factor positive.
[a] Mann Whitney U.
[b] Chi squared.

The authors' studies have confirmed previous reports that UA generally has a better prognosis than RA. Patients with persistent UA had progressive joint involvement and worsening functional disability, but did not seem to require additional DMARD therapy or have significantly progressive erosive disease. Compared with RA patients with similar disease duration, UA patients were less likely to require prednisone or DMARDs, had fewer affected joints, were more likely to be seronegative, were less likely to have radiographic erosions, and had better functional ability, as evidenced by lower modified Health Assessment Questionnaire scores and more full-time employment (Table 5). Predictors of disease persistence could not be determined in this study.

Treatment of early undifferentiated arthritis

It is now widely recognized that early treatment of RA improves clinical outcomes by reducing synovitis and reducing or preventing joint damage and functional disability. Remission or potential cure may be possible if therapy is started early enough to prevent the establishment of self-sustaining pathologic immune processes in the synovium. In RA, DMARDs are initiated much earlier in the course of disease, often in combinations, and a role for biologic agents in very early disease currently is being advocated. The optimal treatment approach for early undifferentiated disease in which a significant proportion spontaneously remit is still unclear, however. Treatment with NSAIDs alone as initial therapy may miss the window of opportunity to intervene in the processes contributing to persistent synovitis, whereas generalized use of potent DMARDs may subject patients to unnecessary potential toxicity. Clinical trials in early disease include only RA patients meeting ACR criteria, and guidelines for therapy in the early UA patient population are hampered by a general lack of clinical data. Treatment-related outcomes reported by at least two early arthritis groups provide some insights, however, into potential appropriate therapeutic approaches.

In the Leeds early arthritis cohort, all patients with clinical synovitis were treated with intramuscular or intra-articular methylprednisolone and reevaluated after 2 weeks as part of the cohort's protocol. DMARDs were considered if the patient progressed to polyarthritis after 12 weeks or if additional corticosteroid treatments were required to the same joints [43,58,59]. As described previously, disease persistence after 6 and 12 months was greater in patients without complete resolution of synovitis within the first few weeks. These findings suggest that early rapid control of synovitis reduces the risk of future progression. Although this finding simply may be due to selecting a milder type of arthritis, it is also possible that rapid treatment may attenuate or abort pathologic immune processes.

The NOAR cohort researchers reported treatment effects on disability and radiographic erosions, while controlling for potential treatment differences using propensity scores. The propensity scores evaluated the likelihood of patients getting treatment based on baseline characteristics, including whether ACR criteria for RA were met [65,66]. Patients were treated at the discretion of their physician. DMARD or corticosteroid use generally was greater in patients with higher indices of disease activity and ultimately meeting criteria for RA; however, a substantial proportion of the cohort was started on treatment before meeting ACR criteria. In their initial report, early treatment improved disability to the level of patients not deemed needing treatment, whereas delayed DMARDs resulted in worse disability [66]. A subsequent study analyzed the proportion of the NOAR cohort who had radiographs (which excluded patients with milder undifferentiated disease) and found that earlier treatment, within 6 months of symptom onset, using conventional DMARDs (most commonly sulfasalazine) or corticosteroids resulted in less radiographic damage than delayed treatment, even in patients without erosions at baseline. This study suggests that early treatment is at least as important as the choice of treatment in early disease, and that sulfasalazine and methotrexate are appropriate first-line therapy [67]. Because a significant proportion of the cohort did not meet ACR criteria for RA at baseline, these findings also may apply to patients with undifferentiated disease, in particular, patients with baseline risks for progression to RA.

Summary

As rheumatologists continue to see patients earlier in the course of their disease, the proportion of patients not meeting standard criteria for specific rheumatologic conditions is likely to increase. In these patients, even more important than assigning a diagnosis is the need to identify patients at risk of developing persistent synovitis, erosive disease, and functional disability, to ensure that appropriate therapeutic measures are initiated. Serologic markers, such as RA-specific autoantibodies (RF, CCP), in combination with clinical features at presentation are the tools are currently available to the clinician for identifying these patients. The most appropriate therapy to choose in UA is unclear and may be less important than prompt control of the inflammatory processes. The duration of therapy and whether therapy can be withdrawn when disease control is achieved also are unknown and need further study. In addition, given the ability to identify RA-specific antibodies in serum years before clinical symptoms are seen, the utility of identifying and treating an at-risk, but asymptomatic population based on autoantibodies is unknown. As knowledge of the basic pathologic events initiating and perpetuating autoimmune synovitis increases and is applied to longitudinal early arthritis cohorts, additional discriminators of disease susceptibility and severity may be identified and provide answers to some of these questions.

References

[1] Lawrence JS, Bennett PH. Benign polyarthritis. Ann Rheum Dis 1960;19:20–30.
[2] Harrison BJ, Symmons DP, Barrett EM, et al. The performance of the 1987 ARA classification criteria for rheumatoid arthritis in a population based cohort of patients with early inflammatory polyarthritis. American Rheumatism Association. J Rheumatol 1998;25:2324–30.
[3] Zeidler H, Merkesdal S, Hulsemann JL. Early arthritis and rheumatoid arthritis in Germany. Clin Exp Rheumatol 2003;21:S106–12.
[4] Wiles N, Symmons DP, Harrison B, et al. Estimating the incidence of rheumatoid arthritis: trying to hit a moving target? Arthritis Rheum 1999;42:1339–46.
[5] Soderlin MK, Borjesson O, Kautiainen H, et al. Annual incidence of inflammatory joint diseases in a population based study in southern Sweden. Ann Rheum Dis 2002;61:911–5.
[6] Savolainen E, Kaipiainen-Seppanen O, Kroger L, et al. Total incidence and distribution of inflammatory joint diseases in a defined population: results from the Kuopio 2000 arthritis survey. J Rheumatol 2003;30:2460–8.
[7] Hernandez-Avila M, Liang MH, Willett WC, et al. Exogenous sex hormones and the risk of rheumatoid arthritis. Arthritis Rheum 1990;33:947–53.
[8] Machold KP, Stamm TA, Eberl GJ, et al. Very recent onset arthritis—clinical, laboratory, and radiological findings during the first year of disease. J Rheumatol 2002;29:2278–87.
[9] Glennas A, Kvien TK, Andrup O, et al. Recent onset arthritis in the elderly: a 5 year longitudinal observational study. J Rheumatol 2000;27:101–8.
[10] Wolfe F, Ross K, Hawley DJ, et al. The prognosis of rheumatoid arthritis and undifferentiated polyarthritis syndrome in the clinic: a study of 1141 patients. J Rheumatol 1993;20:2005–9.
[11] Cunnane G, Grehan S, Geoghegan S, et al. Serum amyloid A in the assessment of early inflammatory arthritis. J Rheumatol 2000;27:58–63.
[12] Soderlin MK, Kautiainen H, Puolakkainen M, et al. Infections preceding early arthritis in southern Sweden: a prospective population-based study. J Rheumatol 2003;30:459–64.
[13] Erlacher L, Wintersberger W, Menschik M, et al. Reactive arthritis: urogenital swab culture is the only useful diagnostic method for the detection of the arthritogenic infection in extra-articularly asymptomatic patients with undifferentiated oligoarthritis. Br J Rheumatol 1995;34:838–42.
[14] Fendler C, Laitko S, Sorensen H, et al. Frequency of triggering bacteria in patients with reactive arthritis and undifferentiated oligoarthritis and the relative importance of the tests used for diagnosis. Ann Rheum Dis 2001;60:337–43.
[15] Schnarr S, Putschky N, Jendro MC, et al. *Chlamydia* and *Borrelia* DNA in synovial fluid of patients with early undifferentiated oligoarthritis: results of a prospective study. Arthritis Rheum 2001;44:2679–85.
[16] Dixey J, Solymossy C, Young A. Is it possible to predict radiological damage in early rheumatoid arthritis (RA)? A report on the occurrence, progression, and prognostic factors of radio-

logical erosions over the first 3 years in 866 patients from the Early RA Study (ERAS).
J Rheumatol 2004;69(Suppl):48–54.

[17] Klarlund M, Ostergaard M, Jensen KE, et al. Magnetic resonance imaging, radiography, and scintigraphy of the finger joints: one year follow up of patients with early arthritis. The TIRA Group. Ann Rheum Dis 2000;59:521–8.

[18] El Gabalawy HS, Goldbach-Mansky R, Smith D, et al. Association of HLA alleles and clinical features in patients with synovitis of recent onset. Arthritis Rheum 1999;42:1696–705.

[19] Jensen T, Klarlund M, Hansen M, et al. Connective tissue metabolism in patients with unclassified polyarthritis and early rheumatoid arthritis: relationship to disease activity, bone mineral density, and radiographic outcome. J Rheumatol 2004;31:1698–708.

[20] van Gaalen FA, Linn-Rasker SP, Van Venrooij WJ, et al. Autoantibodies to cyclic citrullinated peptides predict progression to rheumatoid arthritis in patients with undifferentiated arthritis: a prospective cohort study. Arthritis Rheum 2004;50:709–15.

[21] Higami K, Hakoda M, Matsuda Y, et al. Lack of association of HLA-DRB1 genotype with radiologic progression in Japanese patients with early rheumatoid arthritis. Arthritis Rheum 1997;40:2241–7.

[22] Ostergaard M, Ejbjerg B, Szkudlarek M. Imaging in early rheumatoid arthritis: roles of magnetic resonance imaging, ultrasonography, conventional radiography and computed tomography. Best Pract Res Clin Rheumatol 2005;19:91–116.

[23] Evangelisto A, Wakefield R, Emery P. Imaging in early arthritis. Best Pract Res Clin Rheumatol 2004;18:927–43.

[24] Goldbach-Mansky R, Lee J, McCoy A, et al. Rheumatoid arthritis associated autoantibodies in patients with synovitis of recent onset. Arthritis Res 2000;2:236–43.

[25] Jansen AL, van der Horst-Bruinsma IE, van Schaardenburg D, et al. Rheumatoid factor and antibodies to cyclic citrullinated peptide differentiate rheumatoid arthritis from undifferentiated polyarthritis in patients with early arthritis. J Rheumatol 2002;29:2074–6.

[26] Jansen LM, van Schaardenburg D, van der Horst-Bruinsma IE, et al. The predictive value of anti-cyclic citrullinated peptide antibodies in early arthritis. J Rheumatol 2003;30:1691–5.

[27] Meyer O, Labarre C, Dougados M, et al. Anticitrullinated protein/peptide antibody assays in early rheumatoid arthritis for predicting five year radiographic damage. Ann Rheum Dis 2003;62:120–6.

[28] Vencovsky J, Machacek S, Sedova L, et al. Autoantibodies can be prognostic markers of an erosive disease in early rheumatoid arthritis. Ann Rheum Dis 2003;62:427–30.

[29] Visser H, le Cessie S, Vos K, et al. How to diagnose rheumatoid arthritis early: a prediction model for persistent (erosive) arthritis. Arthritis Rheum 2002;46:357–65.

[30] Vittecoq O, Pouplin S, Krzanowska K, et al. Rheumatoid factor is the strongest predictor of radiological progression of rheumatoid arthritis in a three-year prospective study in community-recruited patients. Rheumatology (Oxf) 2003;42:939–46.

[31] Visser H. Early diagnosis of rheumatoid arthritis. Best Pract Res Clin Rheumatol 2005;19:55–72.

[32] Vossenaar ER, Despres N, Lapointe E, et al. Rheumatoid arthritis specific anti-Sa antibodies target citrullinated vimentin. Arthritis Res Ther 2004;6:R142–50.

[33] Boire G, Cossette P, de Brum-Fernandes AJ, et al. Anti-Sa/citrullinated vimentin antibodies (anti-Sa Abs), anti-cyclic citrullinated peptide (anti-CCP) Abs and IgM rheumatoid factor (RF) as prognostic markers of disease severity in early polyarthritis (EPA) patients. [abstract] Arthritis Rheum 2003;48(9 Suppl):S666.

[34] Vittecoq O, Incaurgarat B, Jouen-Beades F, et al. Autoantibodies recognizing citrullinated rat filaggrin in an ELISA using citrullinated and non-citrullinated recombinant proteins as antigens are highly diagnostic for rheumatoid arthritis. Clin Exp Immunol 2004;135:173–80.

[35] Newkirk MM, Goldbach-Mansky R, Lee J, et al. Advanced glycation end-product (AGE)-damaged IgG and IgM autoantibodies to IgG-AGE in patients with early synovitis. Arthritis Res Ther 2003;5:R82–90.

[36] Berglin E, Padyukov L, Sundin U, et al. A combination of autoantibodies to cyclic citrullinated peptide (CCP) and HLA-DRB1 locus antigens is strongly associated with future onset of rheumatoid arthritis. Arthritis Res Ther 2004;6:R303–8.

[37] van Gaalen FA, van Aken J, Huizinga TW, et al. Association between HLA class II genes and autoantibodies to cyclic citrullinated peptides (CCPs) influences the severity of rheumatoid arthritis. Arthritis Rheum 2004;50:2113–21.

[38] Gough A, Faint J, Salmon M, et al. Genetic typing of patients with inflammatory arthritis at presentation can be used to predict outcome. Arthritis Rheum 1994;37:1166–70.

[39] Harrison B, Thomson W, Symmons D, et al. The influence of HLA-DRB1 alleles and rheumatoid factor on disease outcome in an inception cohort of patients with early inflammatory arthritis. Arthritis Rheum 1999;42:2174–83.

[40] Salmon M, Wordsworth P, Emery P, et al. The association of HLA DR beta alleles with self-limiting and persistent forms of early symmetrical polyarthritis. Br J Rheumatol 1993;32: 628–30.

[41] Vos K, Visser H, Schreuder GM, et al. Human leukocyte antigen-DQ and DR polymorphisms predict rheumatoid arthritis outcome better than DR alone. Hum Immunol 2001;62:1217–25.

[42] Vos K, van der Horst-Bruinsma IE, Hazes JM, et al. Evidence for a protective role of the human leukocyte antigen class II region in early rheumatoid arthritis. Rheumatology (Oxf) 2001; 40:133–9.

[43] Green M, Marzo-Ortega H, McGonagle D, et al. Persistence of mild, early inflammatory arthritis: the importance of disease duration, rheumatoid factor, and the shared epitope. Arthritis Rheum 1999;42:2184–8.

[44] Kvien TK, Glennas A, Melby K. Prediction of diagnosis in acute and subacute oligoarthritis of unknown origin. Br J Rheumatol 1996;35:359–63.

[45] Reece RJ, Canete JD, Parsons WJ, et al. Distinct vascular patterns of early synovitis in psoriatic, reactive, and rheumatoid arthritis. Arthritis Rheum 1999;42:1481–4.

[46] Canete JD, Rodriguez JR, Salvador G, et al. Diagnostic usefulness of synovial vascular morphology in chronic arthritis: a systematic survey of 100 cases. Semin Arthritis Rheum 2003;32: 378–87.

[47] Bresnihan B. Are synovial biopsies of diagnostic value? Arthritis Res Ther 2003;5:271–8.

[48] Hitchon CA, El-Gabalawy HS. The histopathology of early synovitis. Clin Exp Rheumatol 2003;21(Suppl 31):S28–36.

[49] Baeten D, Peene I, Union A, et al. Specific presence of intracellular citrullinated proteins in rheumatoid arthritis synovium: relevance to antifilaggrin autoantibodies. Arthritis Rheum 2001;44:2255–62.

[50] El Gabalawy HS, Hitchon CA, Schumacher HR, et al. Synovial histopathological features and RA autoantibodies predict persistence in patients with synovitis of recent onset. [abstract] Arthritis Rheum 2003;48(9 Suppl):S667.

[51] Harrison B, Symmons D. Early inflammatory polyarthritis: results from the Norfolk Arthritis Register with a review of the literature: II. outcome at three years. Rheumatology (Oxf) 2000; 39:939–49.

[52] Dixon WG, Symmons DP. Does early rheumatoid arthritis exist? Best Pract Res Clin Rheumatol 2005;19:37–53.

[53] Inaoui R, Bertin P, Preux PM, et al. Outcome of patients with undifferentiated chronic monoarthritis: retrospective study of 46 cases. Joint Bone Spine 2004;71:209–13.

[54] Forslind K, Ahlmen M, Eberhardt K, et al. Prediction of radiological outcome in early rheumatoid arthritis in clinical practice: role of antibodies to citrullinated peptides (anti-CCP). Ann Rheum Dis 2004;63:1090–5.

[55] Kastbom A, Strandberg G, Lindroos A, et al. Anti-CCP antibody test predicts the disease course during 3 years in early rheumatoid arthritis (the Swedish TIRA project). Ann Rheum Dis 2004;63:1085–9.

[56] Schumacher Jr HR, Habre W, Meador R, et al. Predictive factors in early arthritis: long-term follow-up. Semin Arthritis Rheum 2004;33:264–72.

[57] Vossenaar ER, Van Venrooij WJ. Anti-CCP antibodies, a highly specific marker for (early) rheumatoid arthritis. Clin Appl Immunol Rev 2004;4:239–62.

[58] Green M, Marzo-Ortega H, Wakefield RJ, et al. Predictors of outcome in patients with

oligoarthritis: results of a protocol of intraarticular corticosteroids to all clinically active joints. Arthritis Rheum 2001;44:1177–83.

[59] Quinn MA, Green MJ, Marzo-Ortega H, et al. Prognostic factors in a large cohort of patients with early undifferentiated inflammatory arthritis after application of a structured management protocol. Arthritis Rheum 2003;48:3039–45.

[60] Jansen LM, van Schaardenburg D, van der Horst-Bruinsma IE, et al. One year outcome of undifferentiated polyarthritis. Ann Rheum Dis 2002;61:700–3.

[61] Tunn EJ, Bacon PA. Differentiating persistent from self-limiting symmetrical synovitis in an early arthritis clinic. Br J Rheumatol 1993;32:97–103.

[62] Raza K, Breese M, Nightingale P, et al. Predictive value of antibodies to cyclic citrullinated peptide in patients with very early inflammatory arthritis. J Rheumatol 2005;32:231–8.

[63] Nissila M, Isomaki H, Kaarela K, et al. Prognosis of inflammatory joint diseases: a three-year follow-up study. Scand J Rheumatol 1983;12:33–8.

[64] Kaarela K. Prognostic factors and diagnostic criteria in early rheumatoid arthritis. Scand J Rheumatol 1985;57(Suppl):1–54.

[65] Bukhari MA, Wiles NJ, Lunt M, et al. Influence of disease-modifying therapy on radiographic outcome in inflammatory polyarthritis at five years: results from a large observational inception study. Arthritis Rheum 2003;48:46–53.

[66] Wiles NJ, Lunt M, Barrett EM, et al. Reduced disability at five years with early treatment of inflammatory polyarthritis: results from a large observational cohort, using propensity models to adjust for disease severity. Arthritis Rheum 2001;44:1033–42.

[67] Hider S, Lunt M, Mottram S, et al. Long-term outcome in inflammatory polyarthritis is not dependent on which disease modifying drug is used first [abstract]. Arthritis Rheum 2004;50:S555.

[68] Woolf AD, Hall ND, Goulding NJ, et al. Predictors of the long-term outcome of early synovitis: a 5-year follow-up study. Br J Rheumatol 1991;30:251–4.

[69] Hall ND, Blake DR, Bacon PA. Serum sulphydryl levels in early synovitis. J Rheumatol 1982;9: 593–6.

[70] Harrison BJ, Symmons DP, Brennan P, et al. Natural remission in inflammatory polyarthritis: issues of definition and prediction. Br J Rheumatol 1996;35:1096–100.

[71] Morel J, Legouffe MC, Bozonat MC, et al. Outcomes in patients with incipient undifferentiated arthritis. Joint Bone Spine 2000;67:49–53.

[72] Mau W, Raspe HH, Mersjann H. Early arthritides: nosography, nosology, and diagnostic criteria. Scand J Rheumatol 1989;79(Suppl):3–12.

[73] Jacobsen S, Madsen HO, Klarlund M, et al. The influence of mannose binding lectin polymorphisms on disease outcome in early polyarthritis. TIRA Group. J Rheumatol 2001;28:935–42.

[74] Nielen MM, van der Horst AR, van Schaardenburg D, et al. Antibodies to citrullinated human fibrinogen (ACF) have diagnostic and prognostic value in early arthritis. Ann Rheum Dis 2005;64(8):1199–204.

[75] Fardellone P, Mejjad O, Vittecoq O, et al. Predictive factors of early radiographic progression in community-recruited patients with very early arthritis: results of the multiparameter prospective VErA study [abstract]. Arthritis Rheum 2003;49(9 Suppl).

[76] Vittecoq O, Pouplin S, Boumier P, et al. Value of clinical and non-clinical parameters for very early diagnosis of rheumatoid arthritis: results of the multiparameter prospective VErA study [abstract]. Arthritis Rheum 2003;49(9 Suppl).

[77] Vittecoq O, Pouplin S, Mejjad O, et al. Predictive factors of persistence of arthritis in the VErA cohort [abstract]. Arthritis Rheum 2003;49(9 Suppl).

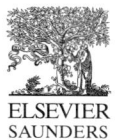

RHEUMATIC
DISEASE CLINICS
OF NORTH AMERICA

Rheum Dis Clin N Am 31 (2005) 627–639

Early Oligoarthritis

Helena Marzo-Ortega, MRCP[a],*, Lorna Cawkwell, MRCP[a],
Michael J. Green, MRCP[a,b,c]

[a]*Academic Unit of Musculoskeletal Disease, Chapel Allerton Hospital, Leeds, UK*
[b]*Harrogate and District NHS Foundation Trust, Harrogate, UK*
[c]*York Hospital, York, UK*

The term oligoarthritis refers to an inflammatory arthritis affecting four or more joints. It is the most common pattern of disease seen in the seronegative arthritides such as reactive arthritis (ReA), psoriatic arthritis (PsA), and inflammatory bowel disease–associated arthritis as well as the group of undifferentiated arthritis [1]. Although rheumatic conditions in general can present with a mono or oligoarticular pattern and subsequently evolve (eg, rheumatoid arthritis), the involvement of less than four joints can significantly narrow the diagnostic possibilities. For example, asymmetric lower limb large joint involvement occurs in ReA, whereas small joints of the fingers, mainly proximal and distal interphalangeal, are typically affected in some subsets of PsA. Oligoarthritis typically affects a young population of patients producing a high level of morbidity [2]. It is a form of arthritis commonly seen in early arthritis clinics [3], yet there are few data on outcome and treatment protocols have not been evaluated. It is the generally held belief that oligoarthritis has a higher chance of remission than polyarthritis, and this has been confirmed with some specific subgroups such as sarcoid arthritis [4]. Likewise, ReA has traditionally been considered to have a good prognosis [5]. However, some studies have reported persistence rates of between 15% and 50% [6], or even as high as 75%, despite the use of disease-modifying antirheumatic drugs (DMARDs) [2].

* Corresponding author. The Academic Unit of Musculoskeletal Disease, Chapel Allerton Hospital, Chapeltown Road, 2nd Floor, Leeds LS7 4SA, UK.
   E-mail address: medhmo@leeds.ac.uk (H. Marzo-Ortega).

Early assessment

As many as 50% of patients with an oligoarthritis may not fulfill a diagnostic criteria at presentation, although it has been suggested that at least one third may have a form of ReA that could have followed an asymptomatic clinical course [7]. A microbiologic assessment should be performed in cases where the clinical history suggests the possibility of recent infection, as it is known that the causative pathogen can be found in 50% of patients presenting with probable or possible ReA [8]. Gastrointestinal and urogenital pathogens may be associated with sterile joint inflammation [9], and evidence of recent infection can be detected either by serology or cultures from the urogenital tract and stool samples in 60% of cases [10]. Enteric infections associated with arthritis include Gram-negative bacteria such as yersinia (mainly *Y enterocolitica,* less so *Y pseudotuberculosis*), salmonella, shigella and campylobacter [11]. Oligoarthritis associated with urogenital infections is most often due to *C trachomatis,* the commonest cause of nongonococcal urethritis. Infection can be silent, particularly in females, so a specific sexual history should be sought, and optimized polymerase chain reaction methods should be applied to first voided early morning urine samples [12]. In addition, specific testing for HIV infection may be indicated as there is a strong association between HIV and the development of spondyloarthritides, in particular ReA and PsA [13,14]. Patients can present with a severe, predominantly lower limb, large joint oligoarthritis in the context of advanced HIV infection, which is largely resistant to antirheumatic treatment. Some reports have suggested resolution of the arthritis with antiretroviral treatment and normalization of CD4 counts [15].

Routine laboratory testing should be performed including inflammatory markers (plasma viscosity, erythrocyte sedimentation rate, or C-reactive protein), which are commonly elevated. Full blood count may show a normocytic normochromic anemia, as may be the case in ankylosing spondylitis (AS) or juvenile arthritis or as a consequence of a persistently elevated acute phase response. In cases of monoarthritis, the differential diagnosis includes: septic arthritis, gout, or crystal arthropathy so serum urate levels and joint aspiration for fluid analysis should be considered. Arthroscopic biopsy may be indicated in cases of diagnostic uncertainty or severe/resistant cases. Hyperuricaemia may however be present in 10% to15% of patients with PsA reflecting overall increased skin activity [16].

Cohort studies in oligoarthritis

When compared with RA, there have been relatively few inception cohort studies examining the outcome of patients presenting with an oligoarthritis of recent onset. Furthermore, due to the number of clinical subsets such as ReA, PsA, and undifferentiated arthritis, there have been many different methods used to define these cohorts with the consequence that the outcome has been variable.

Scatterkirchner and Kruger [17] described a cohort of 119 patients with human leukocyte antigen (HLA)–B27 positive oligoarthritis and demonstrated that 34% of patients were asymptomatic after 2 to 6 years, whereas 25% had evolved into a spondyloarthropathy and over one quarter had disease that relapsed recurrently. The report with the longest period of follow-up came from a study performed in Finland [18], which looked at the 23 year follow-up of 64 patients who presented with an oligoarthritis (defined as four or fewer joints involved) of less than 6 months duration and who were seronegative for rheumatoid factor. From an original cohort of 441 patients with any early inflammatory arthritis, they limited selection for the study to those who had been examined in the outpatient clinic at 8 years follow-up and were still attending. Results showed that only a small minority of patients (n = 3) had to give up their job or finish work due to their arthritis and 15% (7 out of 47) developed radiologic erosions at a mean follow-up of 22 years.

Patients with a definite diagnosis of RA have a better outcome if treated early with DMARDs [19]. The majority of patients with RA are started on therapy when they are first diagnosed. Candidate strategies in managing patients with an early oligoarthritis also include a "watch and wait" policy, which has the disadvantage of missing any opportunity for disease modification, or a blanket therapy with DMARDs to all patients at presentation, which has the disadvantage of ovetreatment in a subgroup of patients with self-limiting disease. On the other hand, corticosteroids allow for a rapid improvement in symptoms demonstrating the reversibility of disease and are widely used in the treatment of oligoarthritis, yet there is a lack of evidence to suggest medium to long-term efficacy.

To address some of these issues, two studies were conducted in Leeds. Subjects were recruited from a dedicated clinic set up in the network context of the Leeds Early Arthritis Clinics. These were the first studies designed to look at the rate of disease persistence in the early stages of an oligoarthritis and to examine the factors predicting persistence in the short- and medium-term. In addition, it was our aim to assess whether early intervention with intra-articular corticosteroids and more latterly a combination approach with intra-articular corticosteroids and sulphasalazine in persistent disease could be used to improve outcome. A total of 110 subjects presenting with disease duration of less than 12 months and who were naïve to either DMARDs or corticosteroids were recruited.

Both cohorts were broadly similar in terms of diagnoses as shown in Table 1. Patients who did not have enough symptoms or signs to satisfy criteria for any specific disease were classified as undifferentiated oligoarthritis; this was the largest subgroup (42%) of which a third had a monoarthritis. The next largest subgroup (24%) were patients with a demonstrable ReA with15% having a genito-urinary infection, 7% enteropathic, and less than 2% poststreptococcal. A minority of patients had RA (12%), PsA (9%), and other diagnoses included irritable bowel disease (IBD)–associated arthritis, sarcoidosis, osteoarthritis, and gout. The first study examined the use of a protocol of intra-articular corticosteroid injections followed by an early review to assess for the presence of persistent synovitis [20]. All synovitic joints were injected in all patients at

Table 1
Breakdown of diagnoses of Leeds oligoarthritis studies

| Diagnoses | Cohort[a] | | | |
| | Green, 2001 [20] | Marzo-Ortega, 2004 [46] | Early oligoarthritis | % |
	(n = 51)	(n = 59)	(n = 110)	
Undifferentiated oligoarthritis (monoarthritis)	24 (6)	22 (9)	46 (15)	42 (14)
ReA	11	15	26	24
Genitourinary	5	11	16	15
Enteropathic	6	2	8	7
Poststreptococcal	0	2	2	<2
Rheumatoid arthritis	8	5	13	12
PsA	6	4	10	9
Undifferentiated SpA	0	6	6	6
IBD arthritis	0	2	2	<2
Sarcoidosis	1	1	2	<2
Osteoarthritis	0	1	1	<1
Gout	1	0	1	<1
Other	0	3	3	<3

[a] First author, year [Ref.].

baseline according to a standard protocol (Table 2). Results showed that at least 50% of patients had a complete response at 2 weeks following the injections, and the best predictor of long-term response at 52 weeks was the presence or absence of synovitis as seen on examination at 2 weeks. Failure to respond by 2 weeks indicated a high likelihood of persistent disease and the need for DMARD therapy. However, despite this good overall initial improvement, 47% of patients had clinical evidence of synovitis at 12 months, indicating a high level of persistence in this young population of patients.

The second study assessed the efficacy of early intervention with intra-articular corticosteroids followed by therapy with sulphasalazine in those patients with persistent or progressive disease and compared it with a group of patients treated with conservative therapy with nonsteroidal anti-inflammatory

Table 2
Dose of intra-articular methylprednisolone recommended for different joints

Joint injected	Dose
Proximal interphalangeal joint	10 mg
Metacarpophalangeal joint	10 mg
Wrist	40 mg
Elbow	40 mg
Shoulder	40 mg
Knee	80 mg
Ankle	40 mg
Metatarsophalangeal joint	10 mg
Interphalangeal joint	10 mg

drugs (NSAIDs) followed by delayed intervention with intra-articular cortico-steroids and sulphasalazine in case of persistent or progressive disease (such as evolution to a polyarthritis). This study was a randomized trial and assessed outcome at 52 weeks in terms of numbers of patients with persistent synovitis and evaluated the impact of treatment on function and work status. Results showed that while both treatment groups demonstrated a reduction in the numbers of patients with synovitis at the primary endpoint, more patients in the early intervention group achieved an absence of synovitis at 1 year (80%) when compared with the conservatively treated group (57%) [21]. In addition, more patients were treated in the first group with sulphasalazine at an earlier stage,

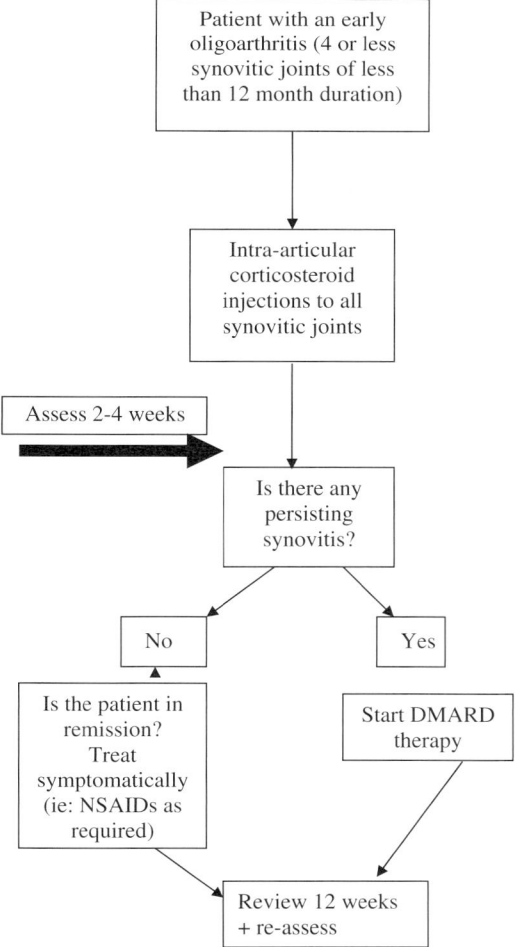

Fig. 1. Suggested guidelines for the management of a patient newly presenting with an oligoarthritis. DMARD, disease-modifying antirheumatic drug; NSAIDs, nonsteroidal anti-inflammatory drugs.

which probably contributed to the positive outcome of the early treated group versus the conservatively treated group, which received both corticosteroids and sulphasalazine at a later stage. The wider use of corticosteroid injections in clinical practice for short-term symptomatic relief is supported by these data, which showed a rapid improvement in pain in the group treated with local injections when compared with the group treated with oral NSAIDs.

The reported rate of persistence of synovitis at 52 weeks in the first study was of 47% [20] which is similar to that of the conservatively treated group (43%) of the second study, and again far in excess of the group that received earlier and more aggressive intervention with corticosteroids and sulphasalazine (20%). A high prevalence of work instability was found in these cohorts with two thirds of patients reporting work impairment at the baseline visits. The long-term outcome is however better with the large majority being able to return to work and maintain their working status by the end of the study [21].

Based on these findings, it is suggested that in early oligoarthritis, all synovitic joints should be injected with intra-articular corticosteroids at presentation and then reassessed soon (eg, 2 to 4 weeks) (Fig. 1). If persistent synovitis is found, DMARDs (eg, sulphasalazine) should be considered without delay or if in remission this could be deferred and the patient observed for a period of time as there is a high chance of long-term remission (H.M.-O., M.J.G., and Anne-Maree Keenan, MAppSC, manuscript in preparation, 2005).

Imaging early oligoarthritis

The evaluation of a patient presenting with oligoarthritis is an important consideration to establish an early diagnosis and to assess effective treatment response. New imaging modalities such as ultrasonography and MRI are changing the way in which early disease is perceived and have in recent years added further information on the primary disease sites and adjacent tissues. These issues are covered more comprehensively elsewhere in this issue and will be discussed here only briefly.

Conventional radiography

Radiography identifies established bone changes and has been the traditional imaging method in rheumatology. Indeed some of the most common oligoarthritic conditions have characteristic structural changes that are identifiable by conventional radiography. For example, marginal erosions can be seen in small peripheral joints in patients with seronegative arthritides as opposed to the central changes seen in rheumatoid arthritis. Distal interphalangeal joint involvement can be seen in PsA as well as osteolysis, pencil-in-cup deformities, or periostitis. In entheseal areas, proliferative new bone formation can be identified particularly in the calcaneum or around the pelvis. Some of these diseases are part of the spectrum of the spondyloarthropathies, whose clinical diagnosis following a different set of criteria hinges heavily in the presence of radiographic sacroiliitis [22,23]. However, most of these changes occur in cases where disease has been present for a number of years and are rarely seen in patients presenting with acute, early oligoarthritis where disease duration may only be weeks or a few months. In these situations, radiography will almost always fail to show any abnormality.

Ultrasound and magnetic resonance imaging

Ultrasound (US) and MRI are rapidly evolving imaging techniques that have advanced our knowledge of the rheumatic process. They are both very sensitive at identifying synovitis and soft tissue pathology. MRI in addition gives detailed information about bone structure. It is this ability to identify early changes in the bone marrow that has allowed in recent years for a better understanding of disease pathogenesis. For example, in RA longitudinal MRI studies show that bone edema precedes the development of bone erosions [24,25] and is associated with the presence of synovitis [24,26]. In the context of seronegative arthritides, MRI has been shown to identify characteristic bone changes in entheseal areas, typical sites of pathology in these diseases both at the peripheral joints [27,28] and the spine [29–31].

US is increasingly used because of its ability to provide information about multiple joints at one examination (and at no extra cost). US is sensitive in the detection of synovitis and bone erosions in small and large joints [32,33]. A recent study in the Leeds cohort of early oligoarthritis patients demonstrated that US is more sensitive than clinical examination for detecting synovitis [34]. Furthermore, US demonstrated that almost two thirds of the patients had evidence of subclinical disease that had not been recognized on clinical examination, while polyarticular disease was seen in another third. These findings have prognostic implications as they confirm that a subset of patients presenting with clinical oligoarthritis in fact represent polyarticular disease in evolution (RA) and may need different treatment. MRI can also demonstrate synovitis in patients with a normal joint examination in early disease. These findings are supported by macro- and microscopic data from arthroscopy in clinically normal knees of patients [35].

Of greatest importance is the fact that these new imaging modalities offer an objective assessment of the extent and severity of disease. Early published evidence has shown a correlation of MRI synovial quantification at baseline with damage at 12 months in RA [24]. More importantly, when synovitis is adequately suppressed, MRI shows reduced bone edema and absence of new lesions over a 3-month period [24]. This short-term benefit is also sustained to 12 months. It therefore appears that adequate suppression of synovitis prevents progression of bone damage. The presence of subclinical synovitis may explain previous reports describing progression of radiographic damage despite what appears to be adequate clinical disease suppression [36]. These results question the sensitivity of clinical examination for detection of low-grade synovitis and therefore whether "early" disease is really that early. Ongoing research in this area may allow for the development of prognostic models as well as genuine' targeted therapeutic regimes. Long-term studies will be required to show a quantitative and qualitative improvement in outcome in order for imaging to be adopted as standard practice.

Treatment of oligoarthritis

Nonsteroidal anti-inflammatory drugs

NSAIDs tend to be the first drugs prescribed after symptom onset and usually before assessment by a rheumatology specialist. NSAIDs can have a dramatic effect on early inflammatory arthritis to the extent of masking the symptoms and signs of inflammatory arthritis. This may offer false reassurance or result in a delay in diagnosis [37]. If there is clinical uncertainty as to the inflammatory nature of a patient's condition, the patient should be reviewed off NSAID therapy: true inflammatory disease will almost certainly deteriorate with NSAID withdrawal and clinical signs may become more apparent. Individual response however can be very varied. In general a long-acting preparation is to be preferred for efficacy, primarily to alleviate prolonged early morning stiffness, with the added benefit of ease of administration, whereas short-acting agents may have advantages for safety.

Intra-articular corticosteroids

Corticosteroids are highly effective in suppressing both COX-2, proinflammatory cytokines and proteases and thus have a number of uses in the management of inflammatory arthritis being used on an induction regimens (before onset of effective DMARD action), in rescue therapy when patients have an acute flare of disease, and at low dosage as part of maintenance therapy. The aim is to use the minimum dose necessary for effective disease suppression without unnecessarily exposing patients to the long-term side effects. Intra-articular corticosteroids can effectively suppress synovitis and are commonly used in the clinic as adjuvant therapy. Local treatment using intra-articular injections has the advantage of delivering a high concentration of corticosteroid to the primary site of pathology. Previous studies in early synovitis have demonstrated that early intervention with intra-articular corticosteroids to all affected joints is associated with prolonged remission [38]. As an inflammatory oligoarthritis has the potential to evolve into a persistent, polyarticular disease such as RA or PsA that in turn can lead to irreversible joint damage, prompt and aggressive intervention with optimal therapies should be initiated and may be truly disease modifying.

Disease-modifying therapies

A number of long-term observational, placebo-controlled trials and delayed therapy studies support the case for early treatment in RA [39]. However, the benefits of early intervention in oligoarthritis have yet to be clearly demonstrated.

The most common subset studied has been that of psoriatic oligoarthritis [40]. It is difficult to draw conclusions as the number of patients included on the different studies is small and trial designs and inclusion criteria differ. Furthermore, these trials are not specific to oligoarthritis and have included patients with predominant axial disease and other clinical patterns.

Sulphasalazine was found to be effective in early disease in spondylarthropathy associated with PsA with clinical and laboratory markers of inflammation improving at 6 months [41]. A randomized, double-blind, controlled trial of sulphasalazine in reactive arthritis showed higher rates inducing remission and early benefit. However this was not maintained beyond 6 months compared with placebo [2]. In a different cohort of PsA patients, follow-up at 36 weeks after treatment with sulphasalazine showed a significant fall in erythrocyte sedimentation rate and a trend toward clinical benefit [40]. There are limited data evaluating the use of methotrexate in the treatment of PsA and again the maximal benefit was seen for early treatment [42]. However, these trials were recruited from established disease populations and extrapolated the data to produce evidence of an early benefit. Also there is little literature on the use of other DMARDs such as leflunomide in oligoarthritic groups.

Further difficulty arises in undifferentiated oligoarthritis, where no trials have been performed despite this being the largest subgroup of oligoarthristis with half the patients remaining "undifferentiated" at 12 weeks. Side effects are not uncommon and a policy of instigating treatment for all patients with early disease will result in individuals who would have had self-limiting disease receiving these drugs. These patients may predominate in specific subgroups of oligoarthritis.

Current evidence suggests that where DMARDs are used, the benefit is maximal in early disease. As there is a high rate of joints requiring re-injection with intra-articular corticosteroids [20], therefore the use of DMARDs in this setting may also be steroid sparing. The question of which DMARD is most effective is still unclear, but sulphasalazine has been the most widely used in trials to date. Likewise it remains to be seen whether response is homogenous in all subgroups of oligoarthritis.

Novel therapies

The advent of biologic therapies in the last decade has heralded a new era in the treatment of arthritis. Drugs that block the action of the pro-inflammatory cytokine tumor necrosis factor (TNF)–α are now licensed for the treatment of inflammatory arthritides such as RA, PsA, and AS and therapies blocking the effect of other cytokines are in various stages of development. Three of these drugs are now approved for patients with RA: the chimeric monoclonal antibody infliximab, the soluble receptor protein etanercept, and the fully humanized monoclonal antibody adalimumab. Infliximab and etanercept have also been shown to be efficacious in spondyloarthropathies, AS, and PsA. So far, no trials have been performed in a large cohort of oligoarthritis patients, although several studies have included a subset of patients presenting with oligoarthritis.

In one study, patients with different spondyloarthropathy subtypes, some of whom had oligoarthritic peripheral joint involvement, were treated with infliximab for a year, during which time response was maintained as shown by parameters of axial and peripheral disease activity [43]. An equivalent response has been seen with etanercept in different subtypes of SpA [29] as well as AS [44]. Several trials have reported the efficacy of these therapies in the treatment of both PsA and skin psoriasis. Although the majority of these reports has included patients with a polyarticular disease pattern, some have included oligoarthritis patients [45] achieving the same level of response with complete resolution of synovitis by 12 weeks as shown by MRI [46]. However, all these studies included patients who had a disease duration greater than 1 year, the majority of whom had well-established disease.

Perhaps, the most exciting development related to the use of these drugs is their ability to halt disease progression. Indeed, some preliminary reports suggest that no radiographic progression was seen in a cohort of patients with established PsA treated with infliximab over a period of 50 weeks [47]. Further data is therefore required from patients treated at earlier stages of disease, where it is postulated there may be a window of opportunity to achieve long-term remission as has been suggested in RA [48].

Antibiotic therapy

The use of antibiotics for the treatment of ReA and undifferentiated oligo-arthritis remains controversial. One of the largest studies to date demonstrated no benefit from a 3-month course of azithromycin in patients with a recent onset (<2 months duration) oligoarthritis (six or fewer joints involved) [49], although there are data suggesting that antibiotics need to be introduced too early in the disease process (before the onset of clinical symptoms) to be of any benefit and that when used late they may increase the length of carriage of bacteria. A recent study has reported possible long-term benefit from a short course of antibiotics in ReA irrespective of the original triggering organism [50]. Previous studies have not been supportive of the use of antibiotics in all patients with an oligoarthritis [51,52] but have suggested some benefit in the enteropathic arthritis subgroup, although this has not been confirmed [53]. Another subgroup that has been studied is that of poststreptococcal ReA where prevention of the progression to a carditis is the main concern. Although data gathered in a controlled fashion is even more sparse than in other subgroups, many advocate the use of prophylactic antibiotics for varying lengths of time of between 1 and 5 years, following the initial symptoms [54].

Summary

Oligoarthritis is a common condition, with a variable outcome, affecting a predominantly young population; when treated conventionally, oligoarthritis has a high morbidity. The variability of outcome has limited the development of studies evaluating therapies such as DMARDs in recent onset disease. Oligoarthritis is an important disease that warrants much greater study.

References

[1] Hübscher O. Pattern recognition in arthritis. In: Klippel JH, Dieppe PA, editors. 2nd edition. Rheumatology, vol. 1. St. Louis (MO): Mosby; 1998. p. 2;3.1–3.6.

[2] Egmose C, Hansen TM, Andersen LS, et al. Limited effect of sulphasalazine treatment in reactive arthritis: a randomized double blind placebo controlled trial. Ann Rheum Dis 1997; 56:32–6.

[3] Parker JD, Capell HA. An acute arthritis clinic—one years experience. Br J Rheumatol 1986; 25:293–5.

[4] Glennas A, Kvein TK, Melby K, et al. Acute sarcoid arthritis: occurrence, seasonal onset, clinical features and outcome. Br J Rheumatol 1995;34(1):45–50.

[5] Toivanen A, Toivanen P. Reactive arthritis. Curr Opin Rheumatol 2000;12(4):300–5.

[6] Fan PT, Yu DTY. Spondyloarthropathies. In: Kelley WN, Harris Jr ED, Ruddy S, Sledge CB, editors. 4th edition. Textbook of rheumatology, vol. 1. Philadelphia: WB Saunders; 1993. p. 59–69.

[7] Schnarr S, Putschky N, Jendro MC, et al. Chlamydia and Borrellia DNA in synovial fluid of patients with early undifferentiated oligoarthritis. Arthritis Rheum 2001;4:2679–85.

[8] Fendler C, Laitko S, Sorensen H, et al. Frequency of triggering bacteria in patients with reactive arthritis and undifferentiated oligoarthritis and the relative importance of the tests used for diagnosis. Ann Rheum Dis 2001;60:337–43.

[9] Leirisalo-Repo M. Enteric infections and arthritis: clinical aspects. In: Calin A, Taurog JD, editors. The spondyloarthropathies. Oxford: Oxford University Press; 1998.

[10] Keat A. Reiter's syndrome and reactive arthritis in perspective. N Engl J Med 1983;309: 1606–15.

[11] Aho K, Leirisalo-Repo M, Repo H. Reactive arthritis. Clin Rheum Dis 1985;11:25–40.

[12] Kuipers JG, Scharmann K, Wollenphaut J, et al. Sensitivities of PCR, Microtrak, Chlamydia EIA, IDEIA, and PACE 2 for purified Chlamydia trachomatis elementary bodies in urine, peripheral blood, peripheral blood leukocytes, and synovial fluid. J Clin Microbiol 1995;33: 3186–90.

[13] Arnett FC, Reveille JD, Duvic M. Psoriasis and psoriatic arthritis associated with human immunodeficiency virus infection. Rheum Dis Clin North Am 1991;17:59–78.

[14] Cuellar ML, Espinoza LR. Human immunodeficiency virus associated spondyloarthropathy: lessons from the third world. J Rheumatol 1999;26:2071–3.

[15] McGonagle D, Reade S, Marzo-Ortega H, et al. Human immunodeficiency virus associated spondyloarthropathy: pathogenic insights based on imaging findings and response to highly active antiretroviral treatment. Ann Rheum Dis 2001;60:696–8.

[16] Espinoza LR, Cuellar ML. Psoriatic arthritis and spondylitis: a clinical approach. In: Calin A, Taurog JD, editors. The spondyloarthropathies. Oxford: Oxford University Press; 1998. p. 97–111.

[17] Scatterkirchner M, Kruger K. Natural course and prognosis of HLA-B27 positive oligoarthritis. Clin Rheumatol 1987;6(Suppl 2):83–6.

[18] Jantti JK, Kaarela K, Lehtinen KES. Seronegative oligoarthritis: a 23 year follow-up study. Clin Rheumatol 2002;21:353–6.

[19] Quinn MA, Conaghan PG, Emery P. The therapeutic approach of early intervention for rheumatoid arthritis: what is the evidence? Rheumatol 2001;40:1211–20.

[20] Green MJ, Marzo-Ortega H, Wakefield RJ, et al. Predictors of outcome in patients with oligo-

arthritis: results of a protocol of intraarticular corticosteroids to all clinically active joints. Arthritis Rheum 2001;44:1177–83.

[21] Marzo-Ortega H, Green MJ, Keenan AM, et al. A randomized trial of intra-articular cortico-steroids versus conservative treatment in early oligoarthritis over 12 months. Arthritis Rheum 2004;50:S198.

[22] Dougados M, van der Linden S, Juhlin R, et al. The European Spondyloarthropathy Study Group preliminary criteria for the classification of spondyloarthropathy. Arthritis Rheum 1991; 34:1218–27.

[23] Amor B, Dougados M, Mijiyawa M. Critères de classification des spondylarthropathies. Rev Rhum 1990;57:85–9.

[24] Conaghan PG, O'Connor P, Mc Gonagle D, et al. Elucidation of the relationship between synovitis and bone damage: a randomised magnetic resonance imaging study of individual joints in patients with early rheumatoid arthritis. Arthritis Rheum 2003;48:64–71.

[25] McQueen FM, Benton N, Perry D, et al. Bone edema scored on magnetic resonance imaging scans of the dominant carpus at presentation predicts radiographic joint damage of the hands and feet six years later in patients with rheumatoid arthritis. Arthritis Rheum 2003;48: 1814–27.

[26] McGonagle D, Conaghan PG, O'Connor P, et al. The relationship of synovitis and bone oedema changes in early untreated rheumatoid arthritis: a controlled magnetic resonance imaging study. Arthritis Rheum 1999;42:1706–11.

[27] McGonagle D, Gibbon W, O'Connor P, et al. Characteristic magnetic resonance imaging entheseal changes in knee synovitis in spondyloarthropathy. Arthritis Rheum 1998;41:694–700.

[28] Jevtic V, Watt I, Razman B, et al. Distinctive radiological features of small hand joint arthritis in rheumatoid arthritis and seronegative spondyloarthritis demonstrated by contrast-enhanced (Gd-DTPA) magnetic resonance imaging. Skel Radiol 1995;24:351–5.

[29] Marzo-Ortega H, McGonagle D, O'Connor P, et al. Efficacy of etanercept in the treatment of the entheseal pathology in resistant spondyloarthropathy. A clinical and magnetic resonance imaging. Arthritis Rheum 2001;44:2112–7.

[30] Braun J, Baralakios X, Golder W, et al. Magnetic resonance imaging examinations of the spine in patients with ankylosing spondylitis, before and after successful therapy with infliximab: evaluation of a new scoring system. Arthritis Rheum 2003;48:1126–36.

[31] Baralakios X, Landewe R, Hermann K-G, et al. Inflammation in ankylosing spondylitis: a systematic description of the extent and frequency of acute spinal changes using magnetic resonance imaging. Ann Rheum Dis 2005;64:730–4.

[32] Wakefield RJ, Gibbon WW, Conaghan PG, et al. The value of ultrasonography in the detection of bone erosion in patients with rheumatoid arthritis: a comaparative study with conventional radiography. Arthritis Rheum 2000;43:2762–70.

[33] Backhaus M, Kamradt T, Sandrock D, et al. Arthritis of the finger joints—a comprehensive approach comparing conventional radiography, scintigraphy, ultrasound, and contrast-enhanced magnetic resonance imaging. Arthritis Rheum 1999;42:232–45.

[34] Wakefield RJ, Green MJ, Marzo-Ortega H, et al. Should oligoarthritis be reclassified? Ultrasound reveals a high prevalence of subclinical disease. Ann Rheum Dis 2004;63:382–5.

[35] Kraan MC, Versendaal H, Jonker M, et al. Asymptomatic synovitis precedes clinically manifest arthritis. Arthritis Rheum 1998;41:1481–8.

[36] Kirwan JR. The relationship between synovitis and erosions in rheumatoid arthritis. Br J Rheumatol 1997;36(2):225–8.

[37] Marzo-Ortega H, Green H, Karim Z, et al. Non-steroidal anti-inflammatory drugs alter the presentation of early inflammatory arthritis. Rheumatol 2000;39(Suppl 1):42.

[38] Devlin J, Gough A, Huisson A, et al. Knee disease in 766 early arthritis patients, relevance to outcome and pathogenesis. Clin Rheumatol 2000;19:82–5.

[39] Quinn MA, Green MJ, Marzo-Ortega H, et al. Prognostic factors in a large cohort of patients with early undifferentiated inflammatory arthritis after application of a structured management protocol. Arthritis Rheum 2003;48(11):3039–45.

[40] Clegg DO, Reda DJ, Mejias E, et al. Comparison of sulfasalazine and placebo in the treat-

ment of psoriatic arthritis. A Depatment of Veterans Affairs Cooperative study. Arthritis Rheum 1996;39(12):2013–20.

[41] Dougados M, van der Linden S, Leirisalo-Repo M, et al. Sulfasalazine in the treatment of spondylarthropathy. A randomized, multicenter, double-blind, placebo-controlled study. Arthritis Rheum 1995;38(5):618–27.

[42] Lacaille D, Stein HB, Raboud J, Klinkhoff AV. Longterm therapy of psoriatic arthritis: intra-muscular gold or methotrexate? J Rheumatol 2000;27(8):1922–7.

[43] Kruithof E, Van den Bosch F, Baeten D, et al. Repeated infusions of infliximab, a chimeric anti-TNF alpha monoclonal antibody in patients with active spondyloarthropathy: one year follow up. Ann Rheum Dis 2002;61:207–12.

[44] Gorman JD, Sack KE, Davis Jr JC. Treatment of ankylosing spondylitis by inhibition of tu-mour necrosis factor alpha. N Engl J Med 2002;346:1349–56.

[45] Mease PJ, Gaffe BS, Metz J, et al. Etanercept in the treatment of psoriatic arthritis and psoria-sis: a randomized controlled trial. Lancet 2000;356:385–90.

[46] Marzo-Ortega H, McGonagle D, Tan AL, et al. A clinical and magnetic resonance imaging assessment of the efficacy of infliximab at a dose of 3 mg/kg in combination with methotrexate in the treatment of psoriatic arthritis. Rheumatol 2004;43(Suppl 2):29.

[47] Antoni C, Kavanaugh A, Gladman D, et al. The infliximab Multinational Psoriatic Arthritis Controlled Trial (IMPACT): results of radiographic analysis after one year. Arthritis Rheum 2004;50:S450.

[48] Quinn MA, Conaghan PG, O'Connor PJ, et al. Very early treatment with infliximab in addi-tion to methotrexate in early, poor-prognosis rheumatoid arthritis reduces magnetic resonance imaging evidence of synovitis and damage with sustained benefit after infliximab withdrawal. Arthritis Rheum 2005;52:27–35.

[49] Kvien TK, Glennas A, Melby K, et al. Reactive arthritis: incidence, triggering agents and clinical presentation. J Rheumatol 1994;21:115–22.

[50] Yli-Kerttula T, Luukkainen R, Yli-Kerttula U, et al. Effect of a three month course of cipro-floxacin on the late prognosis of reactive arthritis. Ann Rheum Dis 2003;62(9):880–4.

[51] Sieper J, Fendler C, Laitko S, et al. No benefit of long term ciprofloxacin treatment in patients with reactive arthritis and undifferentiated oligoarthritis. A three month, multicenter, double blind, randomized, placebo controlled study. Arthritis Rheum 1999;7:1386–96.

[52] Laasila K, Laasonen L, Leirisalo-Repo M. Antibiotic treatment and long-term prognosis of rective arthritis. Ann Rheum Dis 2003;62(7):655–8.

[53] Sieper J, Braun J, Kingsley GH. Report on the fourth international workshop on reactive arthritis. Arthritis Rheum 2000;4:720–34.

[54] Ayoub EM, Majeed HA. Poststreptococcal reactive arthritis. Curr Opin Rheumatol 2000;12:306–10.

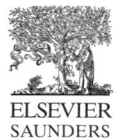
ELSEVIER
SAUNDERS

Rheum Dis Clin N Am 31 (2005) 641–657

RHEUMATIC
DISEASE CLINICS
OF NORTH AMERICA

Early Psoriatic Arthritis

David Kane, PhD, MRCPI[a,b,*], Sanjay Pathare, MRCP(UK)[b]

[a]School of Clinical and Medical Sciences, University of Newcastle-upon-Tyne,
Newcastle-upon-Tyne, UK
[b]Musculoskeletal Department, Freeman Hospital, Newcastle-upon-Tyne, UK

Psoriasis is a common hyperkeratotic skin disease that affects 2% of the population. Psoriatic arthritis (PsA) is an inflammatory arthritis associated with psoriasis that affects peripheral synovial joints and entheses and the axial skeleton [1]. In the past it was considered to be a variant of rheumatoid arthritis (RA) occurring in patients with psoriasis, but it is now recognized as a distinct clinical entity. PsA is estimated to occur in 10% to15% of patients with psoriasis and in early arthritis clinics PsA accounts for up to 13% of patients [2]. Initially PsA was considered to have a benign course, particularly as PsA was usually compared with established RA, and early diagnosis and treatment were not considered a priority by rheumatologists. There is now accumulating evidence that PsA is a chronic, progressive disease that leads to significant joint damage and loss of function with negative impact on quality of life, capacity to work, and life span [3,4]. This has led to the prioritization by rheumatologists for earlier diagnosis and more effective treatment strategies for patients with PsA.

Definition of early psoriatic arthritis

There is still no single accepted definition for PsA. Of the three principal studies of early PsA cohorts, the St. Vincent's University Hospital, Dublin cohort and the University of Padova, Italy cohort have used the Moll and Wright definition [1]. This defines PsA as an inflammatory arthritis associated with psoriasis and usually with negative rheumatoid factor (RF). The Norfolk Arthritis

* Corresponding author. School of Clinical and Medical Sciences, University of Newcastle-upon-Tyne, Framlington Place, Cookson Building, Newcastle-upon-Tyne, NE2 4HH, UK.
E-mail address: d.j.kane@ncl.ac.uk (D. Kane).

Register (NOAR) cohort also applied the Moll and Wright definition but without regard to rheumatoid factor. Fournie and colleagues [5] have reported the only validated criteria for discriminating PsA from RA and ankylosing spondylitis (AS), but these were applied in patients with a mean disease duration of 5 years and they have not been validated in other earlier disease populations. In the early arthritis clinic, a number of problems may arise when applying either Moll and Wright's definition or Fournie and colleagues' classification criteria.

Patients may not be aware of the presence of psoriasis, which can be minimal, and up 20% of patients with PsA do not have psoriasis when they initially develop inflammatory arthritis [6] and may be classified as undifferentiated seronegative arthritis. The features that should alert the clinician to look for psoriasis in a patient are presence of distal interphalangeal (DIP) joint involvement, dactylitis, asymmetric pattern of joint involvement, and nail lesions. Given the high prevalence of psoriasis in the general population a number of patients with other inflammatory arthritis—RA, reactive arthritis, AS, sarcoidosis—may also have psoriasis and be diagnosed inaccurately as PsA, leading to inappropriate treatment. Therefore clinicians must undertake a thorough evaluation of patients with early inflammatory arthritis to detect psoriasis and to rule out other arthritides. Though most patients will have plaque psoriasis on the scalp (Fig. 1) or extensor aspects of limbs and trunk, it is also important to check hidden sites such as the umbilicus, natal cleft, and soles of feet.

Role of rheumatoid factor

Whether one should diagnose PsA or RA in patients with psoriasis and inflammatory arthritis with a positive RF is also controversial. Although most patients with PsA will have a negative RF, the Dublin early PsA cohort included a small number of patients with low positive RF (titers <1:80) [2]. The NOAR

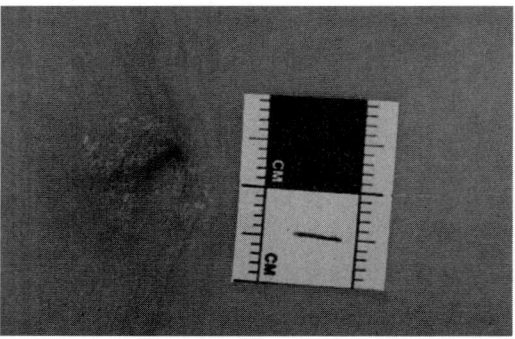

Fig. 1. Plaque psoriasis behind the ear. Although most patients will have plaque psoriasis on the scalp or extensor aspects of limbs and trunk, this can be minimal in psoriatic arthritis. It is also important to check hidden sites such as the umbilicus, natal cleft, and soles of feet. (Courtesy of Lesley Kay, MD, Newcastle-upon-Tyne, UK.)

early PsA cohort included all patients with inflammatory arthritis and psoriasis but 13% were RF positive although the titers were not specified [7] and the Italian cohort did not report RF titers. Clearly the application of the criteria for absent or low RF is important in epidemiologic studies until it is clarified whether PsA patients with RF positivity will have a more severe arthropathy than those who are RF negative. In clinical practice, rheumatologists usually interpret the RF in the context of the clinical features of the arthropathy and the diagnosis of PsA may be considered in patient with psoriasis and inflammatory arthritis and positive RF when the pattern of joint involvement is typical of PsA (eg, dactylitis, DIP joint or spinal involvement, or classic radiologic changes).

The chronologic definition of early PsA has been extrapolated from early RA studies. Early PsA has been defined in two studies as having a disease duration of < 2 years and the cohorts comprise mostly disease-modifying antirheumatic drug (DMARD)-naïve patients [2,7]. In other studies it varies from < 1 year [8] to < 5 years [9]. In the Dublin cohort, it was noted that despite all patients being seen within 2 weeks of referral from their primary care physician, 38% had a disease duration of more than 1 year at first presentation and the 2-year cut-off was deemed appropriate.

Classification of early psoriatic arthritis

PsA is a heterogenous disease that has been subclassified by number (oligoarticular, polyarticular) and pattern (symmetry or asymmetry) of joint involvement in addition to presence or absence of specific features such as spinal involvement, DIP joint involvement, enthesitis, and dactylitis. It has been argued that the degree of symmetry of joint involvement is principally a function of the number of joints involved, which should be given more prominence in PsA classification [10]. A comparison of the different published classification criteria in patients with established PsA and RA found that the criteria of Gladman and colleagues [11], McGonagle and colleagues [12], and Vasey and Espinoza [13] were the most accurate and feasible for distinguishing between PsA and RA [14].

The application of classification criteria in early PsA is further complicated as patients may alter classification as the articular disease evolves. A retrospective evaluation of the presenting patterns of articular disease in 100 patients with established PsA (mean duration = 12.1 years) found that 64% of patients had changed from their pattern at first presentation [15]. A total of 65% of patients with oligoarticular or monoarticular disease had evolved into a polyarticular pattern, whereas only 8% of patients with polyarticular disease had evolved into oligoarticular. In a prospective study of classification in the Dublin early PsA cohort, patients initially classified as having oligoarticular disease were less frequently (23%) reclassified as having polyarticular disease at 2 years [16] and were more likely to be in DMARD–free remission at follow-up. These studies suggest that the number of joints involved at initial assessment has prognostic value, a finding also reported in more established PsA [17].

DIP involvement is a characteristic feature of PsA and DIP-predominant disease was originally described by Moll and Wright [1] as one of five subclasses of PsA but has been given lesser importance in more recent PsA classification criteria [18]. Classification by DIP involvement in the Dublin early PsA cohort was associated with the clinical manifestations of enthesopathy and nail disease but was not useful in predicting clinical or radiologic outcome. In the Italian early PsA cohort no patient was found to have DIP-predominant disease and the NOAR cohort did not differentiate patients by DIP involvement.

Initial attempts to classify early PsA using imaging techniques have produced interesting insights, although the diagnostic and prognostic value of classifying patients by imaging findings is incompletely determined. The plain radiographic pattern at presentation may assist in classifying early PsA as 20% of patients in one study were found to be misclassified when classification was based on clinical assessment alone [19]. Most reclassification of early PsA was due to the identification of spinal involvement—sacroiliitis or syndesmophytes—on plain radiographs at first presentation. MRI studies in spondyloarthropathy (SpA) have identified prominent entheseal inflammation in early disease and have led to proposals for an imaging-based classification of PsA centered on the anatomic localization of disease, although this requires prospective analysis [12].

There is currently no single accepted classification system for early or established PsA [1,6,12,20], and most clinicians usually classify patients for clinical management purposes according to number of joints involved and the presence or absence of enthesitis or spinal disease. Further research is required to determine whether classification criteria are sensitive and accurate in the diagnosis of early PsA, whether they can be used to predict prognosis and outcome, and whether imaging-based classification is more accurate than clinical-based classification.

Epidemiology of early psoriatic arthritis

Analysis of patients with inflammatory arthritis referred to specialist early arthritis clinics suggests that PsA occurs in 5% to 13% of early inflammatory arthritis patients [2,7]. Four U.S.– and Northern European population–based studies report incidence rates of PsA in different populations as ranging from 6 to 8 per 100,000 population [21–24], whereas one study noted an incidence of 3 per 100,000 in Greek patients [25]. The NOAR early arthritis study calculated an incidence of 3.5 per 100,000 [7], and the Dublin early PsA study calculated an incidence rate of 6.7 per 100,000 [2]. Both the NOAR and Dublin studies may underestimate the incidence of PsA as neither included patients with spinal disease alone and the NOAR study estimate did not include patients with oligoarthritis or those who developed psoriasis after the onset of arthritis. The lack of universally accepted diagnostic or classification criteria for PsA and the fact that the majority of epidemiologic studies of PsA are hospital based limits the interpretation of these figures [26]. The estimated prevalence of PsA in the United Kingdom has been calculated as 0.3% using primary care data [27].

Pathogenesis of psoriatic arthritis: insights from early studies

Most existing studies of the pathogenetic mechanisms in PsA do not differentiate early and established PsA patients, and it is not known if similar immunologic and biologic events are occurring at first presentation and in the later, chronic stages of disease. The development of early arthritis clinics and arthroscopic synovial biopsy has facilitated the specific investigation of the earliest stages of PsA. However, patients presenting with PsA to early arthritis clinics still have a median disease duration at presentation of 6 to 7 months [2,7], synovial biopsy is limited to a few specialist centers, and basic research in early PsA is in a development stage. This section reviews insights into PsA pathogenesis and prognosis obtained from research in early PsA patients.

Genetic: human leukocyte antigen and tumor necrosis factor genes

There is considerable evidence that psoriasis and PsA have a genetic predisposition. Associations of susceptibility to PsA with the human leukocyte antigen (HLA) antigens Cw6, B13, B17, and HLA-DR7α have been reported [28–32]. HLA-B27 has been associated consistently with the presence of radiologic sacroileitis but not spondylitis without sacroileitis [33–35], and HLA B38 and B39 are associated with peripheral joint disease [34,36]. There is initial but very limited evidence that HLA genes may have some utility in predicting prognosis in early PsA. HLA DR4 is increased in those with RA-like disease and those with severe arthritis [30,34], and in the University of Toronto cohort HLA antigens B27, B39, and DQw3 were associated with disease progression, whereas HLA-DR7 and B22 were protective [37].

One study has reported that functional tumor necrosis factor (TNF) allele polymorphisms are associated with radiologic outcome in early PsA. In 147 Irish PsA patients, radiologic joint erosion was significantly associated with the TNF-α–308 A ($P \leq .0001$) and TNFB1 ($P = .0009$) alleles [38]. The TNF-α -308 A ($P = .01$) and TNFB1 ($P = .04$) alleles were also increased significantly in a progressor group (19 out of 52 early PsA patients in whom the number of joint erosions in the hands and feet increased over a median interval of 24 months) as compared with the nonprogressor group. These data suggest that high TNF production is associated with the progression of peripheral arthritis in PsA. The potential use of HLA and TNF genes as prognostic markers in the clinical management of early PsA requires further evaluation and remains an area of active research interest.

Environmental: infection and trauma

Because of the well-recognized link between group A streptococcal infection of the throat and the sudden onset of guttate psoriasis, a number of investigators have sought to link streptococcal infection and articular inflammation [39,40]. There is no evidence to suggest a role for routine screening for streptococcal throat infection in early PsA. HIV infection is associated with an increased prevalence of PsA. PsA associated with HIV infection tends to be polyarticular, lower limb predominant, and progressive. The possibility of HIV infection should be considered in patients with early PsA, particularly in individuals with high-risk behavior and in areas of high HIV prevalence.

Patients with early PsA may report preceding musculoskeletal traumatic injury. A controlled study noted that the onset of PsA after trauma in the preceding 3 months was more frequent than was observed in RA and AS [8]. This was associated with higher erythrocyte sedimentation rate and C-reactive protein at presentation and with higher IL-6 levels in the synovial fluid of posttraumatic PsA patients compared with a control PsA group. The investigators postulate that this may be a form of Koebner phenomenon affecting the joint. The clinical evolution of posttraumatic PsA patients was indistinguishable from that of the nontraumatic PsA patients. The progression of early PsA may be influenced by nerve trauma. Several studies point to a lack of inflammatory and radiologic progression of articular diease in PsA in denervated limbs or digits [41–43].

Synovitis and cytokine expression

Synovial inflammation in PsA is characterized by a similar degree of lymphocyte infiltration as is observed in RA, but there is less macrophage infiltration and lining layer hyperplasia with increased vascularity [44]. Synovitis in early PsA has similar features [45], which have been noted as early as 2 weeks disease duration [46] but no study has directly compared the synovitis of early and established PsA. Studies in early PsA have noted increased vascularity and morphogenic changes in synovial blood vessels when compared with RA synovium [47]. These changes are associated with increased vascular endothelial growth factor (VEGF) and matrix metalloprotease (MMP)–9 expression with reduced endothelial apoptosis in the synovium and suggest that further pathogenetic insights may be obtained from studies of synovial vascular endothelium in early PsA.

Increased synovial fluid levels of the proinflammatory cytokines interleukin (IL)-1 β and IL-6 have been reported in early PsA, being higher in patients with elderly onset and posttraumatic PsA [48,49] and in patients with monoarthritis that progressed to involve other joints [49]. The synovial cytokine profile of early PsA has not been examined specifically, although early PsA patients are included in the two largest studies of PsA synovium. These studies note expression of IL-1β, TNF- α, and IL-15 though levels were lower than in RA. TNF-α is also present in psoriasis skin [50] and PsA synovial fluid [51], and a central role for TNF-α in skin and joint inflammation has been been further underlined by the success of TNF inhibition in established PsA [52]. Currently TNF inhibition is used in established PsA, but earlier use in the future in patients with severe PsA and poor prognosis markers is likely.

Clinical presentation

Psoriasis

From analysis of five early PsA cohorts [2,7,15,19,48], the mean disease duration at initial presentation of early PsA has been reported as ranging from 6 to 12 months (Table 1). The median age at onset of psoriasis ranges from 27 to31 years with a median age of PsA onset of 38 in three studies and 52 in the NOAR study. Although an association between severe PsA and moderate to severe psoriasis has been reported in one series of patients with established PsA, there is little evidence of a relationship between the severity of skin and joint disease in early PsA. Nail changes of pitting, horizontal ridging, and onycholysis are specific features of psoriasis that are associated with development of PsA [53] and are present in approximately two thirds of patients with early PsA. Harrison and associates [7] noted that the presence of psoriasis did not influence the presentation or 1 year outcome in patients with early inflammatory polyarthritis, whereas Stafford and colleagues [54] noted that in patients with early SpA, predominantly involving lower limbs, the presence of psoriasis was associated with increased disease persistence and radiologic damage.

Peripheral joint involvement

Peripheral joint involvement in early PsA is more frequent than axial joint involvement, and polyarticular disease is slightly more frequent than oligoarticular disease (see Table 1). The small joints of hands and feet are the most commonly involved peripheral joints [2,7]. Polyarticular onset of PsA is associated with more aggressive disease and with increased progression to joint damage [2]. Polyarticular onset is also associated with older age of arthritis and psoriasis onset, which may be a reflection of the association of elderly onset PsA with more severe inflammatory joint disease [48]. DIP joint involvement is present in 20% to 39% of patients with early PsA and is associated with nail disease but does not associate with different clinical or radiologic outcomes. The DIP predominant pattern of PsA and involvement of the sternoclavicular joints (as in SAPHO syndrome) are rare in early PsA.

Enthesitis and dactylitis

Dactylitis of the fingers and toes or "sausage digit" is a common feature of early PsA being present in approximately one third of patients. Imaging studies have confirmed that dactylitis is principally caused by flexor tenosynovitis and marked adjacent soft tissue swelling with a variable degree of small joint synovitis [55–57]. Enthesitis is defined as inflammation at the site of insertion of tendons and ligaments to the bone and is also a common feature of early PsA. Enthesitis in early PsA is most frequently present at the plantar fascia insertion on calcaneus, achilles tendon insertion, and patellar ligament and quadriceps tendon insertions.

Table 1
Clinical features of early psoriatic arthritis

	First author, year [Ref.]					
	Kane, 2003 [2]	Punzi, 1999 [48][a]		Harrison, 1997 [7]	Jones, 1994 [15][a]	Khan, 2003 [19][a]
Clinical characteristics	(n = 129)	Yo PsA (n = 50)	EoPsA (n = 16)	(n = 51)	(n = 100)	(n = 86)
Sex (M:F)	68:61	23:27	8:8	25:26	43:57	64:36
Median duration arthritis at presentation (y)	0.6	<1	<1	0.5	12.1	0.6
Median age at onset of arthritis (y)	38	44.2	65.1	52	37.6	38.2
Median age at onset of psoriasis (y)	27	—	—	—	28.9	31.1
No. of Swollen joints	4	6.7[b]	12.2[b]	7	6	—
DIP joint involvement (%)	39	—	—	20	27	—
Dactylitis (%)	29	37.5	30	—	—	—
Nail disease (%)	67	—	—	—	67	—
Classification						
Polyarticular (%)	60	—	—	100	25	42
Oligoarticular (%)	40	—	—	0	63	38
Spinal (%)	0	—	—	0	10	20
% remission at 1 y (no. of patients)	26 (31/119)	—	—	6 (3/51)	—	—
HAQ at presentation	0.63	—	—	0.63	0.375	—
HAQ at follow-up	0.13 at 1 y	—	—	0.44 at 1 y	0.5 at 5 y	—
% erosions at presentation (no. of patients)	27 (32/117)	—	—	—	53 (40/75)	—
% erosions at follow-up (no. of patients)	47 at 2 y (40/86)	—	—	22 at 1 y (7/32)	68 at 5 y (51/75)	—

Abbreviations: F, female; HAQ, health assessment questionnaire; M, male.
  [a] Values as means.
  [b] Active joints (either swollen or tender).

Analysis of 401 Italian PsA patients identified 14 patients who had enthesitis and dactylitis as the sole manifestations of PsA [58]. The investigators suggest that this may be an uncommon form of early PsA not recorded by current classification systems and therefore not specifically reported in early PsA cohorts. The incidence of characteristic features of seronegative disease such as dactylitis, nail dystrophy, enthesopathy, and radiologic sacroiliitis are equally distributed in early PsA irrespective of pattern of joint involvement and age of disease onset [2,16,48].

Spinal involvement

Spinal involvement—sacroileitis or spondylitis—in the absence of peripheral joint involvement occurs in only 2% to 4% of patients with established PsA but is present in up to 33% of all patients with established PsA [11] and up to 20% of patients with early PsA [19]. Initially spinal involvement was considered rare in early PsA [59] but two studies from the University of Toronto PsA cohort suggest that spinal involvement may often be clinically silent, requiring plain radiography for diagnosis [19,60]. In another series, radiologic evidence of cervical spine involvement was present in 40 (70%) of 57 patients with PsA, but only 40% had symptoms of inflammatory neck disease [61]. The radiologic pattern of spinal involvement is similar to that observed in AS, although patients with AS have more severe spinal disease, as evidenced by the presence of syndesmophytes and grade 4 sacroiliitis. In PsA spondylitis, men have more severe spinal disease than women [3,62].

Diagnosis and measurement of disease activity in early psoriatic arthritis

The diagnosis of early PsA is usually made on clinical grounds as outlined in the section on the definition of early PsA, but laboratory analyses and imaging studies provide an objective means of confirming the diagnosis and monitoring disease activity.

Acute phase response

The erythrocyte sedimentation rate and C-reactive protein are usually elevated in patients with early PsA and can be used to confirm joint inflammation and to monitor disease activity [2,63]. Although they have not been shown to be individually superior to clinical joint scores, high levels of C-reactive protein are associated with the development of joint damage [63] and a low erythrocyte sedimentation rate is protective for disease progression [64].

Plain radiography

Plain radiography is currently the imaging standard for long-term and medium-term evaluation of disease progression in PsA (Fig. 2). Up to 67% of

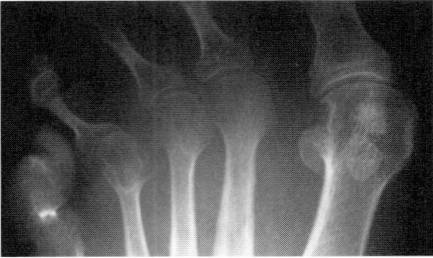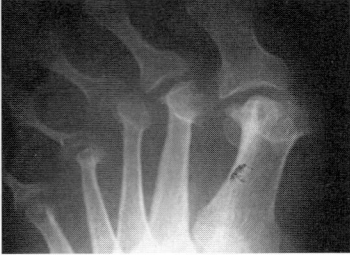

Fig. 2. Plain radiograph of metatarsophalangeal joints at presentation (*left panel*) of PsA and after 2 years of follow-up (*right panel*).

patients with established PsA have radiological manifestations of articular disease [11] that may include soft tissue swelling, erosions, joint space narrowing, periostitis, bony proliferation including enthesophyte formation, periarticular osteoporosis, anklyosis, osteolysis, and joint space widening. In early PsA the most frequent abnormalities are soft tissue swelling, joint erosions, joint space narrowing, and periostitis [2]. Erosions of the joints of the hands and feet in early PsA are similar in morphology to those of early RA, although they tend to be distributed more asymmetrically and may involve DIP joints [2]. Periostitis is a more characteristic feature of PsA than RA and occurs in the metaphyses and diaphyses of bone in early PsA, whereas periarticular osteoporosis is more typically described in early RA. Progression of erosions, bony proliferation, and joint space widening are associated with late and more destructive PsA. The principal roles of plain radiography in early PsA are to rule out other structural pathology, identify more aggressive articular disease, and to establish a baseline to compare future radiographs to in the detection of progression of joint disease.

Four studies have quantified radiographic damage in early PsA. Data from the NOAR study examined 51 cases of early PsA (median disease duration of 6 months) [7]. Plain radiographs of hands and feet were available at 1 year of follow-up in 32 patients and 7 of 32 (22%) demonstrated erosions. In two studies of the St Vincent's University Hospital, Dublin (SVUH) early PsA population, 129 patients (median disease duration of 7 months) were examined. 32 of 117 (27%) had radiographic erosions of hands and feet at presentation increasing to 40 of 86 (47%) at 2 years of follow-up. A separate analysis of all spondylarthropathy patients attending the SVUH early arthritis clinic found that patients with PsA were twice as likely to have joint erosions of hands and feet as patients with reactive arthritis and undifferentiated SpA [65]. Punzi [66] did not report the frequency of joint damage in early PsA but noted that erosions are more frequent in the hands than in the feet in early PsA.

The mean rate of radiologic damage is slow in early PsA. The SVUH cohort reported that the mean modified (to include DIPs) Sharp erosion score at presentation was 1.2 increasing to 3 at 2 years. The frequency of joints with erosions was low increasing from 2.1% to 3.9% in the hands and from 2.2% to 6.2% in the feet. In a cohort of 50 Italian patients with early PsA (disease duration

< 1 year, age < 60) the mean and standard deviation number of erosions in hands was 2.2 ± 2.2 at presentation and 2.7 ± 2 after 1 year [66]. In this study, the rate of progression of erosions was higher in the feet over 1 year and greater in a comparator group of patients with early PsA over 60 years of age. The SVUH cohort did not demonstrate any difference in Sharp score related to age, although periostitis was only observed in patients under the age of 60.

Spondylitis and sacroiliitis may also occur in early PsA and the radiographic appearances are similar to those of early AS, although plain radiography is relatively insensitive for early inflammatory disease of the spine and MRI is more specific and sensitive.

Musculoskeletal ultrasound

High-resolution ultrasonography (US) has been validated as a sensitive technique in the detection of synovitis in established PsA [67] with one report finding it to be superior to MRI [68]. Extensive evaluation of the technique has been performed in early RA where US has been demonstrated to be more sensitive than clinical examination in the detection of synovitis and joint effusion [69,70]. These studies have not been reproduced in early PsA, although in the authors' practice, US is widely used to diagnose synovitis and monitor response to therapy in early PsA.

US is more sensitive than clinical examination in diagnosing enthesitis in PsA although the published data do not discriminate between early and established PsA [71,72]. US provides higher resolution of tendon and ligament infrastructure than MRI and allows real-time clinical assessment of any abnormalities identified. Additionally US examination of enthesitis has revealed that new bone formation in the enthesis is present in PsA and not RA [73].

Power Doppler is a technique that allows identification of low-velocity blood flow as occurs in inflamed synovium and entheses. Again this has been validated in the diagnosis of synovitis [67] and enthesitis [72,74] in established PsA but not specifically in early PsA. A single study has noted that power Doppler signal is only observed in enthesitis associated with SpA such as PsA and not in RA, which may assist in diagnosis at early stages of PsA [72].

In early RA, US and MRI have been proven to be more sensitive than plain radiography in the detection of joint erosions. Though US has great potential to be used in the detection of bone erosion in early PsA, this has yet to be validated. However, if US and MRI are proven to be more sensitive than plain radiography in the detection of bony erosion in early PsA, they have the potential to replace plain radiography as the gold standard. This is particularly the case in clinical trials where the difference in the rates of damage progression may be very small in active treatment limbs [52].

Magnetic resonance imaging

MRI allows high-definition imaging of soft tissues cartilage and bone with a wider field of view than standard ultrasound. MR and US have similar indications in the detection of synovitis, enthesitis, and erosions in early PsA, although use of MRI is limited by its availability and expense. Extrapolation of experience from early RA suggests that it is likely to be as sensitive and specific in the diagnosis of joint synovitis and bony erosion in early PsA, although this remains to be confirmed. In early SpA patients, including patients with early PsA, with hand and knee inflammation, MR revealed prominent extracapsular entheseal-associated abnormalities that were significantly less frequent in RA [75]. This suggested a role for MR in the differential diagnosis of early PsA and early RA though this remains to be proven.

Computed tomography

CT has been found to be superior to plain radiography but not to US and MRI in the detection of early humeral bone erosions in RA, and CT is inferior to US and MRI in the diagnosis of synovitis [76]. As CT involves ionizing radiation, US and MRI are generally preferred for evaluating joints in early inflammatory arthritis, including PsA. CT and MRI are comparable in the imaging of chronic sacroiliitis, although MR is superior in early sacroiliitis and in spondylitis as MRI is capable of imaging subchondral and bony edema, an early feature of active sacroiliitis and spondylitis.

Scintigraphy

Nuclear scintigraphy is useful in the diagnosis of early synovitis [68] and in the detection of sacroiliitis [66] in early PsA although MR and ultrasound are usually preferred.

Management of early psoriatic arthritis

Evidence from early RA suggests that the early diagnosis and treatment of inflammatory arthritis can produce better outcome in terms of damage and function [77]. With increasing awareness of the outcome of early PsA, the approach of early diagnosis and treatment has been adapted to the management of PsA. Though this approach seems appropriate, there are limited data on the effectiveness of this strategy and limited evidence of efficacy for most DMARDs in PsA. There is a clear need for comparative studies of DMARDs in early and established PsA that would address this deficit of information.

Nonsteroidal anti-inflammatory drugs (NSAIDs) are usually used for immediate symptom control in most patients with a greater use of DMARDs now occurring in the early stages of PsA. Sulphasalazine and methotrexate are the two commonest DMARDs used in early PsA [2]. Both are effective in peripheral joint disease but sulphasalazine does not improve spondylitis or skin disease [78–81]. Methotrexate, leflunomide, and cyclosporine are effective in ameliorating skin and peripheral joint disease but have no effect on spinal inflammation [82,83] with the effects of methotrexate and cyclosporine in combination producing an additive improvement [84]. Of the other DMARDs, azathioprine appears to have benefit in treating peripheral synovitis with no effect on skin and spine disease [85]. Intra-articular corticosteroids are effective whereas oral corticosteroids are generally avoided because of the risk of rebound flare of psoriasis on withdrawal of steroids.

TNF inhibition with either etanercept [52] or infliximab [86] has proven beneficial in the management of peripheral synovitis and psoriasis and in the management of spondylitis [87]. The management of early inflammatory arthritis is dealt with more comprehensively in the chapters on DMARDs and biologic therapy.

Summary

Studies of early and established PsA confirm that most patients with PsA have persistent inflammation, develop progressive joint damage and disability, and have reduced life expectancy [2,4,88]. Patients with RA and PsA who are matched for age, sex, and duration of disease have comparable radiologic severity [89]. Only 12% of patients with early PsA will be in DMARD–free remission at 2 years [16]. Whereas 18% of patients with established PsA experience remission at some point during the course of their disease, half of these will relapse. These data have lead to a change in clinical practice with the emphasis now on earlier diagnosis and more intensive treatment of patients with PsA. The introduction of biologic therapy provides clinicians with a treatment that finally targets all three sites of disease in the PsA: the skin, synovium, and enthesis. Long-term follow-up of cohorts who receive early diagnosis and intensive treatment are required to demonstrate that this approach will translate into improved outcomes for patients with PsA.

References

[1] Moll JMH, Wright V. Psoriatic arthritis. Semin Arthritis Rheum 1973;3:55–78.
[2] Kane D, Stafford L, Bresnihan B, FitzGerald O. A prospective, clinical and radiological study of early psoriatic arthritis: an early synovitis clinic experience. Rheumatology (Oxford) 2003;42(12):1460–8.
[3] Gladman DD. Natural history of psoriatic arthritis. Baillieres Clin Rheumatol 1994;8(2): 379–94.
[4] Gladman DD, Farewell VT, Wong K, Husted J. Mortality studies in psoriatic arthritis: results from a single outpatient center. II. Prognostic indicators for death. Arthritis Rheum 1998;41(6): 1103–10.
[5] Fournie B, Crognier L, Arnaud C, et al. Proposed classification criteria of psoriatic arthritis. A preliminary study in 260 patients. Rev Rhum Engl Ed 1999;66(10):446–56.
[6] Veale D, Rogers S, FitzGerald O. Classification of clinical subsets in psoriatic arthritis. Br J Rheumatol 1994;33(2):133–8.

[7] Harrison BJ, Silman AJ, Barrett EM, et al. Presence of psoriasis does not influence the presentation or short-term outcome of patients with early inflammatory polyarthritis. J Rheumatol 1997;24(9):1744–9.

[8] Punzi L, Pianon M, Bertazzolo N, et al. Clinical, laboratory and immunogenetic aspects of post-traumatic psoriatic arthritis: a study of 25 patients. Clin Exp Rheumatol 1998;16(3): 277–81.

[9] Harrison BJ, Hutchinson CE, Adams J, et al. Assessing periarticular bone mineral density in patients with early psoriatic arthritis or rheumatoid arthritis. Ann Rheum Dis 2002;61(11): 1007–11.

[10] Helliwell PS, Hetthen J, Sokoll K, et al. Joint symmetry in early and late rheumatoid and psoriatic arthritis: comparison with a mathematical model. Arthritis Rheum 2000;43(4): 865–71.

[11] Gladman DD, Shuckett R, Russell ML, et al. Psoriatic arthritis (PSA)—an analysis of 220 patients. Q J Med 1987;62(238):127–41.

[12] McGonagle D, Conaghan PG, Emery P. Psoriatic arthritis: a unified concept twenty years on. Arthritis Rheum 1999;42(6):1080–6.

[13] Vasey FB, Espinoza LR. Psoriatic arthropathy. In: Calin A, editor. Spondyloarthropathies. New York: Grune and Stratton; 1984. p. 151–85.

[14] Taylor WJ, Marchesoni A, Arreghini M, et al. A comparison of the performance characteristics of classification criteria for the diagnosis of psoriatic arthritis. Semin Arthritis Rheum 2004;34(3):575–84.

[15] Jones SM, Armas JB, Cohen MG, et al. Psoriatic arthritis: outcome of disease subsets and relationship of joint disease to nail and skin disease. Br J Rheumatol 1994;33(9):834–9.

[16] Kane D, Stafford L, Bresnihan B, FitzGerald O. A classification study of clinical subsets in an inception cohort of early psoriatic peripheral arthritis—'DIP or not DIP revisited'. Rheumatology (Oxford) 2003;42(12):1469–76.

[17] Gladman DD, Farewell VT. Progression in psoriatic arthritis: role of time varying clinical indicators. J Rheumatol 1999;26(11):2409–13.

[18] Veale D, FitzGerald O. Psoriatic arthritis–"DIP or not DIP? That is the question." Br J Rheumatol 1992;31(6):430–1.

[19] Khan M, Schentag C, Gladman DD. Clinical and radiological changes during psoriatic arthritis disease progression. J Rheumatol 2003;30(5):1022–6.

[20] Torre Alonso JC, Rodriguez Perez A, Arribas Castrillo JM, et al. Psoriatic arthritis (PA): a clinical, immunological and radiological study of 180 patients. Br J Rheumatol 1991;30(4): 245–50.

[21] Isomaki H, Raunio J, von Essen R, Hameenkorpi R. Incidence of inflammatory rheumatic diseases in Finland. Scand J Rheumatol 1978;7(3):188–92.

[22] Kaipiainen-Seppanen O. Incidence of psoriatic arthritis in Finland. Br J Rheumatol 1996; 35(12):1289–91.

[23] Shbeeb M, Uramoto KM, Gibson LE, et al. The epidemiology of psoriatic arthritis in Olmsted County, Minnesota, USA, 1982–1991. J Rheumatol 2000;27(5):1247–50.

[24] Soderlin MK, Borjesson O, Kautiainen H, et al. Annual incidence of inflammatory joint diseases in a population based study in southern Sweden. Ann Rheum Dis 2002;61(10):911–5.

[25] Alamanos Y, Papadopoulos NG, Voulgari PV, et al. Epidemiology of psoriatic arthritis in northwest Greece, 1982–2001. J Rheumatol 2003;30(12):2641–4.

[26] Veale DJ. The epidemiology of psoriatic arthritis: fact or fiction? J Rheumatol 2000;27(5): 1105–6.

[27] Kay LJ, Parry-James JE, Walker DJ. The prevalence and impact of psoriasis and psoriatic arthritis in the primary care population in the North East England. Arthritis Rheum 1999; 42:S299.

[28] Armstrong RD, Panayi GS, Welsh KI. Histocompatibility antigens in psoriasis, psoriatic arthropathy, and ankylosing spondylitis. Ann Rheum Dis 1983;42(2):142–6.

[29] Woodrow JC, Ilchysyn A. HLA antigens in psoriasis and psoriatic arthritis. J Med Genet 1985;22(6):492–5.

[30] Gladman DD, Anhorn KA, Schachter RK, Mervart H. HLA antigens in psoriatic arthritis. J Rheumatol 1986;13(3):586–92.

[31] Murray C, Mann DL, Gerber LN, et al. Histocompatibility alloantigens in psoriasis and psoriatic arthritis. Evidence for the influence of multiple genes in the major histocompatibility complex. J Clin Invest 1980;66(4):670–5.

[32] Espinoza LR, Vasey FB, Oh JH, et al. Association between HLA-BW38 and peripheral psoriatic arthritis. Arthritis Rheum 1978;21(1):72–5.

[33] Brewerton DA, Caffrey M, Nicholls A, et al. HL-A 27 and arthropathies associated with ulcerative colitis and psoriasis. Lancet 1974;1(7864):956–8.

[34] Gerber LH, Murray CL, Perlman SG, et al. Human lymphocyte antigens characterizing psoriatic arthritis and its subtypes. J Rheumatol 1982;9(5):703–7.

[35] Marsal S, Armadans-Gil L, Martinez M, et al. Clinical, radiographic and HLA associations as markers for different patterns of psoriatic arthritis. Rheumatology (Oxford) 1999;38(4):332–7.

[36] Beaulieu AD, Roy R, Mathon G, et al. Psoriatic arthritis: risk factors for patients with psoriasis - a study based on histocompatibility antigen frequencies. J Rheumatol 1983;10(4):633–6.

[37] Gladman DD, Farewell VT. The role of HLA antigens as indicators of disease progression in psoriatic arthritis. Multivariate relative risk model. Arthritis Rheum 1995;38(6):845–50.

[38] Balding J, Kane D, Livingstone W, et al. Cytokine gene polymorphisms: association with psoriatic arthritis susceptibility and severity. Arthritis Rheum 2003;48(5):1408–13.

[39] Vasey FB, Deitz C, Fenske NA, et al. Possible involvement of group A streptococci in the pathogenesis of psoriatic arthritis. J Rheumatol 1982;9(5):719–22.

[40] Muto M, Date Y, Ichimiya M, et al. Significance of antibodies to streptococcal M protein in psoriatic arthritis and their association with HLA-A*0207. Tissue Antigens 1996;48(6):645–50.

[41] Veale D, Farrell M, FitzGerald O. Mechanism of joint sparing in a patient with unilateral psoriatic arthritis and a longstanding hemiplegia. Br J Rheumatol 1993;32(5):413–6.

[42] Mulherin D, Bresnihan B, FitzGerald O. Digital denervation associated with absence of nail and distal interphalangeal joint involvement in psoriatic arthritis. J Rheumatol 1995;22(6): 1211–2.

[43] Kane D, Lockhart JC, Balint PV, et al. Protective effect of sensory denervation in inflammatory arthritis (evidence of regulatory neuroimmune pathways in the arthritic joint). Ann Rheum Dis 2005;64(2):325–7.

[44] Veale D, Yanni G, Rogers S, et al. Reduced synovial membrane macrophage numbers, ELAM-1 expression, and lining layer hyperplasia in psoriatic arthritis as compared with rheumatoid arthritis. Arthritis Rheum 1993;36(7):893–900.

[45] Reece RJ, Canete JD, Parsons WJ, et al. Distinct vascular patterns of early synovitis in psoriatic, reactive, and rheumatoid arthritis. Arthritis Rheum 1999;42(7):1481–4.

[46] Kane D, Gogarty M, O'Leary J, et al. Reduction of synovial sublining layer inflammation and proinflammatory cytokine expression in psoriatic arthritis treated with methotrexate. Arthritis Rheum 2004;50(10):3286–95.

[47] Fraser A, Fearon U, Reece R, et al. Matrix metalloproteinase 9, apoptosis, and vascular morphology in early arthritis. Arthritis Rheum 2001;44(9):2024–8.

[48] Punzi L, Pianon M, Rossini P, et al. Clinical and laboratory manifestations of elderly onset psoriatic arthritis: a comparison with younger onset disease. Ann Rheum Dis 1999;58(4): 226–9 [see comments].

[49] Punzi L, Bertazzolo N, Pianon M, et al. Value of synovial fluid interleukin-1 beta determination in predicting the outcome of psoriatic monoarthritis. Ann Rheum Dis 1996;55(9):642–4.

[50] Ritchlin C, Haas-Smith SA, Hicks D, et al. Patterns of cytokine production in psoriatic synovium. J Rheumatol 1998;25(8):1544–52.

[51] Partsch G, Wagner E, Leeb BF, et al. T cell derived cytokines in psoriatic arthritis synovial fluids. Ann Rheum Dis 1998;57(11):691–3.

[52] Mease PJ, Goffe BS, Metz J, et al. Etanercept in the treatment of psoriatic arthritis and psoriasis: a randomised trial. Lancet 2000;356(9227):385–90.

[53] Scarpa R, Oriente P, Pucino A, et al. Psoriatic arthritis in psoriatic patients. Br J Rheumatol 1984;23(4):246–50.

[54] Stafford L, Kane D, Murphy E, et al. Psoriasis predicts a poor short-term outcome in patients with spondylarthropathy. Arth Care Res 2001;45:485–93.

[55] Olivieri I, Barozzi L, Favaro L, et al. Dactylitis in patients with seronegative spondylarthropathy. Assessment by ultrasonography and magnetic resonance imaging. Arthritis Rheum 1996; 39(9):1524–8.

[56] Olivieri I, Barozzi L, Pierro A, et al. Toe dactylitis in patients with spondyloarthropathy: assessment by magnetic resonance imaging. J Rheumatol 1997;24(5):926–30.

[57] Kane D, Greaney T, Bresnihan B, et al. Ultrasonography in the diagnosis and management of psoriatic dactylitis. J Rheumatol 1999;26(8):1746–51.

[58] Salvarani C, Cantini F, Olivieri I, et al. Isolated peripheral enthesitis and/or dactylitis: a subset of psoriatic arthritis. J Rheumatol 1997;24(6):1106–10.

[59] Lambert JR, Wright V. Psoriatic spondylitis: a clinical and radiological description of the spine in psoriatic arthritis. Q J Med 1977;46(184):411–25.

[60] Hanly JG, Russell ML, Gladman DD. Psoriatic spondyloarthropathy: a long term prospective study. Ann Rheum Dis 1988;47(5):386–93.

[61] Salvarani C, Macchioni P, Cremonesi T, et al. The cervical spine in patients with psoriatic arthritis: a clinical, radiological and immunogenetic study. Ann Rheum Dis 1992;51(1):73–7.

[62] Gladman DD, Brubacher B, Buskila D, et al. Psoriatic spondyloarthropathy in men and women: a clinical, radiographic, and HLA study. Clin Invest Med 1992;15(4):371–5.

[63] Helliwell PS, Marchesoni A, Peters M, et al. Cytidine deaminase activity, C reactive protein, histidine, and erythrocyte sedimentation rate as measures of disease activity in psoriatic arthritis. Ann Rheum Dis 1991;50(6):362–5.

[64] Gladman DD, Farewell VT, Nadeau C. Clinical indicators of progression in psoriatic arthritis: multivariate relative risk model. J Rheumatol 1995;22(4):675–9.

[65] Stafford L, Kane D, Murphy E, et al. Psoriasis predicts a poor short-term outcome in patients with spondylarthropathy. Arthritis Rheum 2001;45:485–93.

[66] Punzi L, Pianon M, Rossini P, et al. Clinical and laboratory manifestations of elderly onset psoriatic arthritis: a comparison with younger onset disease. Ann Rheum Dis 1999;58(4):226–9.

[67] Fiocco U, Cozzi L, Rubaltelli L, et al. Long-term sonographic follow-up of rheumatoid and psoriatic proliferative knee joint synovitis. Br J Rheumatol 1996;35(2):155–63.

[68] Backhaus M, Kamradt T, Sandrock D, et al. Arthritis of the finger joints: a comprehensive approach comparing conventional radiography, scintigraphy, ultrasound, and contrast- enhanced magnetic resonance imaging. Arthritis Rheum 1999;42(6):1232–45.

[69] Szkudlarek M, Court-Payen M, Jacobsen S, et al. Interobserver agreement in ultrasonography of the finger and toe joints in rheumatoid arthritis. Arthritis Rheum 2003;48(4):955–62.

[70] Karim Z, Wakefield RJ, Quinn M, et al. Validation and reproducibility of ultrasonography in the detection of synovitis in the knee: a comparison with arthroscopy and clinical examination. Arthritis Rheum 2004;50(2):387–94.

[71] Balint PV, Kane D, Wilson H, et al. Ultrasonography of entheseal insertions in the lower limb in spondyloarthropathy. Ann Rheum Dis 2002;61(10):905–10.

[72] D'Agostino MA, Said-Nahal R, Hacquard-Bouder C, et al. Assessment of peripheral enthesitis in the spondylarthropathies by ultrasonography combined with power Doppler: a cross-sectional study. Arthritis Rheum 2003;48(2):523–33.

[73] Frediani B, Falsetti P, Storri L, et al. Ultrasound and clinical evaluation of quadricipital tendon enthesitis in patients with psoriatic arthritis and rheumatoid arthritis. Clin Rheumatol 2002; 21(4):294–8.

[74] Balint PV, Sturrock RD. Inflamed retrocalcaneal bursa and Achilles tendonitis in psoriatic arthritis demonstrated by ultrasonography. Ann Rheum Dis 2000;59(12):931–3.

[75] McGonagle D, Gibbon W, O'Connor P, et al. Characteristic magnetic resonance imaging entheseal changes of knee synovitis in spondylarthropathy. Arthritis Rheum 1998;41(4):694–700.

[76] Alasaarela E, Suramo I, Tervonen O, et al. Evaluation of humeral head erosions in rheumatoid arthritis: a comparison of ultrasonography magnetic resonance imaging, computed tomography and plain radiography. Br J Rheumatol 1998;37(11):1152–6.

[77] Emery P. The Roche Rheumatology Prize Lecture. The optimal management of early rheumatoid disease: the key to preventing disability. Br J Rheumatol 1994;33(8):765–8.

[78] Fraser SM, Hopkins R, Hunter JA, et al. Sulphasalazine in the management of psoriatic arthritis. Br J Rheumatol 1993;32(10):923–5.

[79] Combe B, Goupille P, Kuntz JL, et al. Sulphasalazine in psoriatic arthritis: a randomized, multicentre, placebo-controlled study. Br J Rheumatol 1996;35(7):664–8.

[80] Farr M, Kitas GD, Waterhouse L, et al. Treatment of psoriatic arthritis with sulphasalazine: a one year open study. Clin Rheumatol 1988;7(3):372–7.

[81] Clegg DO, Reda DJ, Mejias E, et al. Comparison of sulfasalazine and placebo in the treatment of psoriatic arthritis. A Department of Veterans Affairs Cooperative Study. Arthritis Rheum 1996;39(12):2013–20.

[82] Cuellar ML, Espinoza LR. Methotrexate use in psoriasis and psoriatic arthritis. Rheum Dis Clin North Am 1997;23(4):797–809.

[83] Kaltwasser JP, Nash P, Gladman D, et al. Efficacy and safety of leflunomide in the treatment of psoriatic arthritis and psoriasis: a multinational, double-blind, randomized, placebo-controlled clinical trial. Arthritis Rheum 2004;50(6):1939–50.

[84] Fraser AD, van Kuijk AW, Westhovens R, et al. A randomised, double-blind, placebo controlled, multi- centre trial of combination therapy with methotrexate plus cyclosporin in patients with active psoriatic arthritis. Ann Rheum Dis 2005;64(6):859–64 [2004].

[85] Jones G, Crotty M, Brooks P. Psoriatic arthritis: a quantitative overview of therapeutic options. The Psoriatic Arthritis Meta-Analysis Study Group. Br J Rheumatol 1997;36(1):95–9.

[86] Antoni C, Krueger GG, de Vlam K, et al. Infliximab improves signs and symptoms of psoriatic arthritis: results of the IMPACT 2 trial. Ann Rheum Dis 2005;64(8):1150–7.

[87] Braun J, Sieper J. Biological therapies in the spondyloarthritides—the current state. Rheumatology (Oxford) 2004;43(9):1072–84.

[88] Gladman DD, Stafford-Brady F, Chang CH, et al. Longitudinal study of clinical and radiological progression in psoriatic arthritis. J Rheumatol 1990;17(6):809–12.

[89] Rahman P, Nguyen E, Cheung C, et al. Comparison of radiological severity in psoriatic arthritis and rheumatoid arthritis. J Rheumatol 2001;28(5):1041–4.

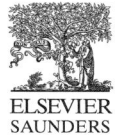

ELSEVIER
SAUNDERS

RHEUMATIC
DISEASE CLINICS
OF NORTH AMERICA

Rheum Dis Clin N Am 31 (2005) 659–679

Early Rheumatoid Arthritis

Adam Young, MD, FRCP*

City Hospital, St. Albans, Herts, UK

Much clinical research in rheumatology involves comparisons of different interventions for specific conditions, the cornerstone being the randomized controlled trial (RCT). If well designed and conducted rigorously, this is the least likely method to introduce bias or false results (grade-A evidence) [1]. However, admission to clinical trials can be and usually is highly selective, and not all clinical research questions can be answered this way. Rheumatoid arthritis (RA) tends to be chronic and can last for decades. It is extremely difficult to retain patients in randomized clinical trials for longer than 2 to 3 years. Obtaining information on the course and outcomes of RA in this way is a major problem. Predicting these outcomes can be important for targeting therapies toward those patients likely to fare badly. The only way to develop reliable prognostic markers and define relevant clinical outcome measures for chronic disease is from inception cohorts with long-term follow-up (grade-B evidence). If well designed and performed to a high standard to reduce bias, longitudinal observational studies can be pivotal in providing information needed for the successful management of chronic disease, and often complement the results of RCTs [2,3]. Prognostic factors that identify patients at risk of more severe disease would allow timely intervention at earlier stages.

Clinical effectiveness of management of rheumatoid arthritis

Identifying the optimal management of RA remains the most important challenge for clinical rheumatology. Although much progress has been made in the last two decades in defining the course of RA, and in the development of new

* City Hospital, St. Albans, Waverly Road, Herts AL3 5PN, UK.
E-mail address: Adam.young@whht.nhs.uk

drugs, outcome in RA remains disappointingly poor. Evidence-based information on disease-modifying antirheumatic drugs (DMARDs), either as sequential monotherapy or combination therapy, has been provided by randomized studies in the short-term (≤ 2–3 years) only. Evidence suggests that the most important phase is the first 12 to 24 months [4]. In recent years there has been a favorable reappraisal of the systematic collection of long-term observational outcomes for chronic diseases like RA [5–7]. Several reports have provided important information on long-term clinical effectiveness of disease-modifying drugs in RA [8–10]. Such studies provide information that RCTs cannot, namely outcomes in true-to-life clinical settings in the medium to long-term. Around half of early RA patients may be excluded from or drop out during RCTs because of restrictions based on age, child-bearing risk, comorbidity, and concurrent drug therapy, logistics, or convenience. This selection bias may have a significant impact on outcome, and although such trials are important for efficacy and adverse events, they often have less bearing on clinical effectiveness. It is the details of the latter that are required at both individual and strategic levels of service planning by patients, clinicians, health authorities, and the pharmaceutical industry, especially in the long-term (Box 1).

The optimal treatment for early RA at present depends on the use of best clinical practice/guidelines currently available, translating results of randomized studies and observational cohorts into routine clinical practice, and defining and identifying patients with poor prognostic factors and poor responses to initial therapies. Problems with this arise firstly because current good clinical practice is known to vary, but little is known about actual practices performed. Secondly, the highly selective, controlled nature and limited length of RCTs do not always relate to ordinary clinical settings. Finally, prognostic factors need further refinement before they can be used in a standardized way routinely in ordinary clinical settings. In an evidence- and cost-based review of rational use of new and existing disease modifying agents, Kremer's guidance [11] was centered on the initial use of methotrexate, which could be followed by sulphasalazine alone or with hydroxychloroquin, then leflunamide or biologics. Similarly, European rheumatologists recommended both the use of at least two DMARDs (one being methotrexate) and persistent disease activity, based on the disease activity score (DAS28), before biologics should be considered [12].

Box 1. Rationale for inception cohort studies with long-term follow up in rheumatoid arthritis

1. Clinical effectiveness of RA management
2. Reflect true-to-life ordinary settings
3. Less selection bias if well-designed
4. Long-term outcomes

Longitudinal observational inception cohort studies in rheumatoid arthritis

Valuable information on the natural (but treated) history of early RA has been provided by a number of inception cohorts. These have been designed essentially to examine the course of RA outside clinical trial settings, using established outcome measures at early (1–3 years), medium (5–7 years) and long-term (≥ 10 years) points and to investigate prognostic factors for these. The clinical, laboratory, and radiologic features of RA during the early years are interesting and have provided insights in the etiology and pathogenesis of this condition. Their more immediate and practical use is monitoring response to therapy. There is a growing body of evidence from these studies that the course of RA is established early. If disease-modifying therapy is to achieve its maximum potential, it must do this before irreversible damage occurs. Thus many inception cohorts have also attempted to develop prognostic factors at early stages to assist clinicians in management decisions within ordinary clinical settings. A number of physician- and patient-centered outcome measures have been developed to achieve this.

Several reviews on early RA studies and predictive features for severity of RA have been published in recent years [13–15]. The main outcomes addressed include functional disability, radiologic change, and mortality. The larger studies have been able to report on the less common or more complicated outcomes of early RA like clinical remission, work disability, and orthopedic interventions. Possible sources of bias in all these studies arise as a result of sample sizes too small for adequate follow-up, left censoring (milder RA not being referred to primary or secondary care), right censoring (more severe RA not surviving long enough for follow-up), and treatment effects. The assessment of drug treatment effects is limited in observational studies because of nonrandom assignment of therapy. Newer agents can only be described as disease-modifying if they can be shown to alter objective measures like radiologic damage in the long-term. The cohorts established to date will permit a comparison of new drugs with well described historic standards reflecting management and costs of RA before the biologic era (Box 2).

Box 2. Requirements for inception cohorts

1. Rigorous data collection
2. Full and unbiased enrolment
3. Subject retention
4. Maximal follow-up
5. Statistical analysis
    a. Use of all data
    b. Account for subject loss

Table 1
Early rheumatoid arthritis inception cohorts with long-term and observational outcomes in chronologic order

Center (location), year started [Ref.]	No. of patients in study	Symptom duration to entry (y)	Followup (y)	Outcomes reported	Measures defined	Additional variables	Prognostic factors at baseline	Predictive power (P value, OR, % classified correctly)
RNHRD (Bath, UK), 1960 [18,87]	100	<1	3–25	F, M	FG	—	FG	$P<0.01$
Middlesex Hospital (London, UK), 1965 [17,20,21,42–44,67,83]	100–149	<1	3–15	Rad, F, M, Rem	Lawrence, FG	HLA-DR4, cervical spine radiographs	RF, Hb, platelet count FG Radiographs	70%–79%
University Hospital (Memphis, TN), 1970 [19]	50	<1	3–5	Rad (hands only)	Erosions	—	RF, joint score, Raynaud, malaise, white race, females	80% (in 3 categories)
Soviet-Finnish (Heinola, Finland), 1980 [105,106]	200–275	<6 mo	6–20	F, Rad	FG, Larsen	—	CRP, ESR Joint scores, RF, grip strength, radiographs, ESR	$P<0.001$ 43% (EV)
University Hospital (Lund, Sweden), 1985 [31,57,68,72,84,100]	100–183	<2	2, 5, 10	F, Rad, WD, M, O, Rem	HAQ, Larsen	HLA-DRB1, SE	HAQ, grip strength HAQ, sex, SE	67%–80% OR 13.4 75%
University Medical Centre (Nijmegen, The Netherlands), 1985 [29,32,33]	147–186	<1	2–10	F, Rad. Com, M	HAQ, Sharp	DA, HLA-DR	RF, HLA DR, DAS, Sharp	83%

University Hospital (Gronigen, The Netherlands), 1985 [41,101]	149	<1	2–10	F, Rad, Com, M	HAQ, Sharp	DA, HLA-DR	RF, HLA DR, CRP, Sharp	46% (EV)
ERAS–9 Centres (UK), 1986 [39,54,58,61,71,86]	745–1064	<2	3, 5, 10	F, WD, Rad, O, M	FG/HAQ, Larsen, all surgery	DA, SE, HLA-DRB1, extra-articular RA	HAQ & SE HAQ & manual work RF & Larsen ESR, Hb, Larsen, & HLA Sex, HAQ, ESR, Hb, Larsen, & SE	78% 90% (1 y) OR 4–5
Leiden University (Leiden, The Netherlands), 1985 [34]	132[a]	<5 (mean 1.6)	6, 12	Rad, F, DA	Kellgren, HAQ, Joint score	HLA typing	Radiographs, IgM & IgG RF, agalactosyl IgG, joint scores, HAQ	70%–80% 76%–78%
Norfolk Arthritis Registrar (NOAR, Norfolk, UK) 1989 [49,59,70,78,88]	175–528	<1	3, 5	F, Rad, M, Rem	HAQ, Larsen	HLA-DRB1, SE	RF, disease duration >3 mo, 2 swollen large joints	71%–80%
Multicenter (Paris & Montpellier, France), 1993 [46,60]	191–800	<1	3, 5	Rad, F	Sharp, HAQ	HLA-DRB1, DAS	ESR, RF, radiographs, HLA HAQ, pain, DAS, radiographs	90+% PPV=93% NPV=46%
Rheumatism Research Centre (Berlin, Germany), 1995 [107]	139	<2	3	Radiographs	Ratingen	HLA-DRB1	HLA, RF, DAS	84%

Abbreviations: Com, comorbidity; DA, disease activity; EV, explained variance; F, function; M, mortality; O, orthopedic; Rad, radiology; Rem, remission; SE, socioeconomic; WD, work disability.

[a] Women only.

What has been learned from these studies that was not apparent from clinical experience, cross-sectional reports, or clinical trials? Is it possible to use prognostic indices generated from these studies in ordinary clinical practice? This article reviews genuine and dedicated inception cohort studies published in mainstream rheumatologic journals, which fulfill the criteria for reporting on longitudinal observational studies [16] and have included clinically relevant and long-term outcomes. The emphasis is on early RA studies rather than reports of symmetrical and undifferentiated polyarthritis or early undiagnosed synovitis. The main studies are shown in Table 1.

The first of these were single hospital-based studies started in the 1960s, two in the UK [17,18] and one in the United States [19]. They all reported on the early course and outcome of RA patients treated with NSAIDs alone, or with Gold injections, d-penicillamine, hydroxychloroquin, and steroids in 50 to150 patients over 3 to 15 years. At this time not all clinical, laboratory, and radiologic assessments were standardized and validated, so comparisons between these, and future studies, are difficult. However, these studies did show that the early course of RA fluctuates a great deal, so much so that it became apparent that the very mild, even remitting form of early RA challenged the accepted diagnostic criteria for RA. These studies reported prodromal symptoms and the pattern of joint involvement at presentation in some detail, which highlighted the importance of foot involvement early on, both clinically [20] and radiologically [21]. Despite this, neither clinical nor radiologic involvement of feet is included in the modified American College of Rheumatology (ACR) criteria for diagnosis of RA [22]. A subgroup of erosive patients was identified in whom no new erosions developed nor progressed after about 3 years [21]. Radiologic assessments available at this time centered around erosions [23] rather than other features of radiologic damage subsequently developed that are more sensitive to change (Box 3) [24,25].

At the same time the two UK studies highlighted for the first time early functional loss, using the same method [26], and the relationship between poor function at presentation and subsequent functional disability. It became apparent that clinical activity measures stabilized or improved but function deteriorated despite DMARD monotherapy. Because of multifactorial influences affecting functional ability, predicting functional outcome with any clinical utility was not achieved then and still remains a problem [14]. On the other hand, predicting

---

Box 3. Findings from first inception cohorts

- Early fluctuating course
- Subgroup with remission or nonprogressive radiographs by 3 years
- Erosions appear more commonly first in feet
- Early reduced function associated with later functional disability

radiologic outcome has always been easier. The UK studies managed to maintain long-term follow-up (ie, > 10 years), but by this stage analysis was hampered by small numbers because of the initial sample sizes. Subsequent to, and based on these initial studies, several other inception cohorts have been assembled, mainly in northern Europe, which have reported on larger numbers of patients and have used validated and standardized assessments, including patient-reported outcomes (eg, health assessment questionnaire [HAQ] [27], short form–36 [SF36] [28]), disease activity scores [DASs] [29], genetics, and radiologic scoring methods. These studies reflect clinical practice after the mid 1980s, namely earlier referral to secondary care and more intensive treatment with a wider range of antirheumatic drugs. Most include, and in fact contributed to, the core data set agreed for these sorts of studies by rheumatology consensus groups [30]. Outcomes have been extended to include the newer technologies like MRI and bone density measurement, socioeconomic tools, and more patient-centered measures like psychosocial assessment, work disability, orthopedic interventions, and comorbidities. In addition, more robust and sophisticated statistical analyses were used. The use of odds ratios (ORs) in univariate analysis and logistic regression in multivariate analysis to demonstrate risk or predictive factors allows these tools to be applied to clinical practice. Table 1 shows the main genuine inception cohorts of RA, which have used standardized assessments, before use of DMARDs, and with at least 3 years observational follow-up in patients on conventional therapies.

Radiologic changes

Most studies have used the Lawrence/Kellgren, Larsen, or Sharp methods to score plain radiographs of hands and feet. Despite this and variations in selection criteria, reported radiologic damage at baseline in most inception cohorts is similar at around 30%. Important findings from the first studies were first involvement only of feet in 36%, compared with hands only (16%), and 48% of erosive patients did not progress after 3 years [21]. This latter figure was higher than the 26% erosive RA who did not progress over 5 years reported from a Swedish cohort [31]. Many of these findings were largely confirmed in the Nijmegen/Groningen study of 147 patients started in the 1980s [32]. After 3 years, 70% had radiographic damage (Sharps method), all of whom could be identified by 1 year. Biannual radiographs showed that the rate of progression was highest in the first year with flattening of the curve in the next 2 years [33], whereas the study from Leiden (Kellgren/Lawrence method) in 135 women showed a linear increase over 6 years [34]. An accelerated phase between 2 and 3 years (Larsen method) has been reported over 5 years [35]. In contrast to these, a community-based study of inflammatory joint disease reported that of 185 patients who developed erosions using Larsen's method, only 66% did so by 2 years, and patients continued to develop erosions after 3 years [36]. Of the patients who had serial radiographs in a study from Wichita, a constant rate of damage over time was seen for all components of Sharps method [37]. Thus, although several different types and rates of radiologic progression have been described, including linear, curvilinear, fast-slow, slow-fast, sigmoid curves [38], erosions or not at 3 years was very similar at around 70%. When the other nonerosive criteria for radiologic change described by Larsen were included, only 14% had normal radiographs at 3 years [39]. The rate of radiologic damage is an important factor in decisions concerning use of disease-modifying drugs.

Although detailed studies have now shown that damage occurs early in plain radiographs [33], the advent of MRI has revealed that changes can be detected even earlier, and erosion of periarticular bone can be present but not apparent on plain films of hands and feet [40]. The erosive process is taking place elsewhere of course and one study described changes taking place in large joints at early stages of RA, with 20% having some damage in at least one joint by 1 year [41]. The first signs of cervical spine damage also start at an early stage [42] and these correlate closely with radiograph progression in hands and feet [43].

Baseline clinical and laboratory measures have been used to predict radiologic outcome with univariate analysis, and most of these studies are consistent in reporting initial radiograph scores, rheumatoid factor (RF), and acute phase reactants as predictors of radiologic damage by around 3 years. However, the reliability and strength of these prognostic markers vary considerably [14]. Other baseline features have had variable success, including articular indices, disease activity scores, various established and novel laboratory measures, and genetic markers. RF alone has been reported to predict erosions or not in 70% [44], and using regression methods, a combination of various independent clinical, laboratory, and genetic factors have achieved better classification (80%–90%) in a number of reports [34,37,39,44–46]. The only consistent baseline prognostic factors from these reports were initial radiograph scores and RF. Disease activity as a laboratory measure (erythrocyte sedimentation rate or C-reactive protein) or a composite score featured in many, and prediction was better using 1-year variables [39]. The role of human leukocyte antigen (HLA)-DRB1 genes remains controversial. Despite many investigators reporting positive, but varying degrees of association of HLA-DRB1*04 RA-associated alleles with radiologic damage [32,34,45,46], others have questioned their predictive value [44,47–49]. Many other laboratory measures with predictive value for radiograph changes have been described in these inception cohorts over the years but have never achieved routine use in clinical settings, mainly because they add little power to the current risk factors available and also because of cost. They are largely covered by the recent review of Kim and Weisman [15] and include serologic markers like IgG and IgA RF, agalactosyl IgG, antikeratin, antiperinuclear, anti-Sa, anti-RA33 and type II collagen antibodies, and metalloproteinase. The extra power provided by these additional serologic and genetic variables is usually disappointingly modest when applied to the clinical setting. Anticyclic citrullinated peptide (anti-CCP) antibodies, however, may have a place [50]. The best for predicting radiologic severity in terms of assisting clinicians with therapeutic decisions early on are still routine measures, which have not changed

---

Box 4. Radiologic progression

- Erosions in ~30% at presentation
- ~70% by 3 years
- Rheumatoid factor and baseline radiograph scores best predictors up to 90%
- Variables at 1 year better predictors
- HLA-DRB1 has doubtful prognostic value

---

much in 30 years, but are now standardized and better applied. At least clinical utility is approached with more than 90% accuracy, with positive and negative predictive values having potential as clinically useful tools [14]. It is not known how much this information is being used in routine practice and although these prognostic factors may not be used formally, it is likely they are part of the judgments made before using disease-modifying drugs or biologic agents (Box 4).

Functional ability

All currently used health status measures have adequate properties in terms of reliability, validity, and responsiveness to change and no doubt will improve with time [51–53]. Their importance is not confined to quality of life issues and clinical trials of new therapies, but also their ability to predict other outcomes, for example work disability [54,55] and mortality [56]. Drawbacks are lack of dimensions for psychologic influence and functional objectivity.

For functional ability, most inception cohort studies have fortunately either used the 4-point scale for functional grade (FG) [26] or the Stanford HAQ disability index [27], so comparisons are possible. These studies have shown wide variation [14], especially in the FG scale, which lacks sensitivity to change between FGII and III but has been largely superseded by the HAQ. The inception cohorts reporting on this have found a wide range of HAQ at presentation but remarkable uniformity in aggregated data, with a mean or median of around 1 (range 0.8–1.3) [57–60]. Although most studies have shown an overall improvement in HAQ over the next few years, there is variation in the rate of change in HAQ. At 2 years 10% of 147 patients [32] and 29% of a community-based study (n = 277) had an HAQ >1 [59]. Combe and associates [60] reported 27% of 191 patients had HAQ >1 at 3 years and 22% at 5 years. Equivalent figures in the ERAS cohort were 34% and 38%, respectively [61]. Explanations for this variation in HAQ values later on in RA include treatment effects and the influence of certain covariates that affect function with time, for example socioeconomic status. Older women from more deprived backgrounds did not follow the normal pattern of improvement in HAQ over 3 years [61].

It has proved much more difficult to predict functional outcome than radiologic changes. In a review of this subject [14], certain features were more notable for their absence, for example female sex, acute phase (erythrocyte sedimentation rate, C-reactive protein) and RF, all of which are generally considered poor prognostic factors but not always so for function. Most studies found that measures of function at early stages predicted functional ability later in disease. These observations were found even in a short-term study of 95 patients at 1 year [62]. Results at 1 year, or changes over the first year expressed as time-integrated measures (area under the curve analysis) [63], were better than at baseline (ie, first visit). Although cumbersome to perform and less useful for early treatment strategies, these more detailed analyses of cumulative effects may produce more meaningful results [64]. A recent survey to determine the use of health status measures in clinical practice reported that the HAQ was most commonly used and was being used to identify problems and monitor disease progression outside research settings [65]. Opinion was divided about the clinical value of these measures, but at least there is consistency in that HAQ in the first year provides some predictive value for later functional ability.

Educational status was first described as one of the most useful predictors of outcome in cross-sectional studies from the United States [66]. Poor socio-economic environments have been shown to effect outcome adversely in many chronic disorders. Whether this feature adds anything to standard clinical or laboratory variables in European countries is still uncertain, because although a relationship with functional outcome has been demonstrated in RA [57,61] there is no agreement concerning its use in clinical settings.

The early studies in the 1970s and 1980s reported associations between early features and eventual functional ability, the strengths of any relationships being based on the size of the P value. More recent reports present results as relative risks (given as an OR), intuitively easier for clinicians to understand. More sophisticated statistical tools have been used to classify patients into two (and sometimes three) outcome groups using the most powerful combination of available baseline variables, which individually may not be useful. The majority of both types of analysis have reported initial functional measures as the most important single predictors of eventual functional ability, but with limited clinical value on an individual patient basis. One report concluded that the observed variance of the baseline HAQ was insufficient to explain the 2-year HAQ [32]. In general combined features performed better than single variables, and modest improvements in prognosis were reported when various other clinical and laboratory indices were combined with measures of function at baseline, with articular indices, sex, RF, erythrocyte sedimentation rate, and hemoglobin featured most commonly. One study examining only standard laboratory tests reported that the performance of RF alone had no value but in combination with hemoglobin and platelet count did achieve modest predictive value for functional outcome [67]. The advantage of classifying patients into the correct versus incorrect group (rather than explained variance) allows the clinician to view the relative performance of baseline variables in predicting favorable versus unfavorable outcomes,

---

Box 5. Functional impairment

- HAQ ≤ 1 in 50% at presentation
- Initial improvement, then gradual deterioration
- Best predictor is baseline function, but only 70%–80% correct
- Associated with increased work disability and mortality
- Not strongly directly-related to radiographs, but
  predicts progression

---

and the relative value of a positive versus a negative predictive value. In general, a poor functional outcome has been easier to predict than a good one. Correctly classifying two outcome groups in this way has improved to 70%–80% of patients, and although still probably not good enough for individual clinical decisions, is the best at present for function. The initial HAQ is almost universally the most powerful predictor, with variation in the value of other variables. Despite this, clinicians should consider the important early indices summarized here, but only in conjunction with the other presenting features which are so critical and specific to each individual patient (Box 5).

Work disability

Permanent work disability has considerable impact on patients' lives, family income, and indirect costs for society. Information important for planning future health care services includes greater detail concerning reasons for loss of or changes in employment during the first few years of RA, regional variations, and whether early recognition and any remedial interventions can be effective. Few inception cohorts have reported on job status, partly because only around 50% of patients are in paid employment when they develop RA [54], thus halving the number of the cohort for analysis. Frequencies for work disability in studies of differing designs from several countries vary from 29% to 50%. Most prospective studies have reported physically demanding jobs and severity of RA as important risk factors for work loss. This was a consistent finding, in spite of the differences in study designs, varying health care and social security arrangements in countries studies, and different methods for ascertaining work disability as entirely due to or only partially due to RA. Work loss occurs early, is generally high at ~30%–40% by 5 years [54,68–70], continues to increase mainly due to RA or comorbidity [54], and it is uncommon for patients to return to work. It can have serious and far-reaching individual, social and economic consequences even within a year or two. Predictors at baseline include worse HAQ at baseline and manual work, a subject that has been reviewed across all types of RA studies [55]. In a regional comparison study in the UK, a combination of HAQ, manual work, erythrocyte sedimentation rate, sex, age, and radiograph erosions predicted work disability correctly in 78% [54]. An important finding from another UK study [70] was lack of evidence that earlier intervention with second-line drugs reduced work disability rates. The results of all these early RA studies should prompt rheumatology departments to identify this problem early in clinical practice and introduce mechanisms to assist patients rather than awaiting public or social services before patients have actually lost their jobs.

Orthopedic surgery

In the last 20 years, orthopedic interventions have no longer been regarded as "last ditch" or salvage surgery, and because of the success of what are now standard and routine procedures like hip, knee, and elbow replacements, their use early on are definite options in the management of RA. In a large inception cohort of over 1000 patients, 12% required some form of surgery for RA within 5 years of presentation, total hip and knee surgery accounting for 7% [71]. The median time to actual surgery was 40 months from baseline, although planned around 6 months earlier. By 10 years, 22% had required surgery. These figures reflect practice in the nationalized UK health service, and surgery for purely for degenerative joint disease was accounted for. Comparisons with other reports are not easy because only a few inception cohorts have reported their findings and sample sizes have been small [72], or study designs have been longitudinal and observational but not from onset or cross-sectional [45,73–75]. These studies report similar figures for surgery rates (7%–10%, 20%, and 25% by 5, 10, and 20 years, respectively) and highlight the occurrence of severe joint failure that may occur within a few years from the onset of RA, despite early use of conventional medical therapy. Both high erythrocyte sedimentation rate and low hemoglobin at 1 year were more strongly associated with large joint replacement surgery than at baseline (with ORs of 4–5), but it was not possible to predict with any accuracy the need for surgery early on using multivariate analysis [71]. Hemoglobin does not normally perform well as a predictor for severity in RA, but has been reported in another study on orthopedic surgery [73]. Women, high swollen joint counts, and Larsen scores were associated with hand and foot surgery, required in 4% by 5 years and in 10% by 10 years. The value of HLA-DRB1 typing varies a great deal. In some retrospective studies, the predictive value of HLA-DRB1 is high; 60% of RA patients that were homozygous for the disease epitope eventually needed a joint replacement in a tertiary referral center in the United States, compared with 25% heterozygote [45], and in secondary care in West Scotland, patients homozygous for the shared epitope (SE) were five times more likely to require major surgery within 15 years [74]. Of the two inception cohorts, patients homozygous for SE were nearly two [71] and three times [72] more likely to require surgery. In contrast to this, a retrospective study of 300 French patients failed to demonstrate any relationship [76]. Apart from study design, interaction with covariates may be an explanation for these discrepancies. In an early RA study from the Netherlands, patients expressing

> **Box 6. Other outcomes**
>
> *Work disability*
>   Occurs in ~30%–40% by 5 years
>   Associated with high baseline HAQ and manual work
>
> *Orthopedic surgery*
>   Occurs in 10%, 20%, and 25% by 5, 10, and 20 years, respectively
>   Variable risk factors (eg, HLA-DRB1, hemoglobin (Hb), erythrocyte sedimentation rate at 1 year)

HLA-DR1 and -DR4 had higher disease activities but yielded no additional information after correcting for RF positivity [77]. If biologic agents have greater disease-modifying properties compared with DMARDs in the long-term, we should see a reduction in orthopedic surgery rates with time (Box 6).

Mortality

Mortality studies have differed considerably in actual mortality rates for both early and established RA, the effects of sex on this, and whether any excesses result from specific conditions, particularly cardiovascular causes. The different study designs (inception, prospective but not early RA or cross-sectional studies, clinic-based or population cohorts) and variations in sample sizes, follow-up periods, and geographic areas may explain some of these differences and why standard mortality ratios (SMR) vary from 149 to 308 in cross-sectional studies [78–81], and from 87 to 140 in RA inception cohorts [82–86]. In addition, treatment practices have changed over the years of study, with increased and early referral to secondary care, earlier use of DMARDs, especially methotrexate, and greater emphasis on tighter disease control. There has been a relative paucity of reports from inception cohorts, and most have limited numbers or follow-up. The two UK-based studies in the 1960s, which both had good follow-up although small sample sizes, reported modest increases in mortality [83,87]. In contrast, two RA inception cohorts started in the late 1980s in northern Europe reported no increase in mortality [84,85]. ERAS started in the UK at much the same time and had very similar study design to these but reported a modest increase in all cause mortality over a maximum 18-year follow-up (median 9 years) in 1415 patients [86]. This increased SMR was restricted to the first 7 years of disease and was largely due to early deaths from cardiovascular in both sexes. Two recent community and primary care cohorts, which generally recruit milder RA, have reported increased mortality in women even in the early years of RA [88,89], with cardiovascular causes prominent very early on [88].

The inception cohort approach may be responsible for some of the variations reported, rather than improved survival in RA [90]. It does allow study of a wider spectrum of RA and is more likely to retain patients with definite but milder disease, some of whom achieve prolonged remission. This reflects more accurately the varied severity and prognosis in RA. Retrospective studies may well be biased toward the more severe patients who would be more likely to be retained in the clinic setting, partly because of comorbidity.

The causes of death in patients with RA are similar to that of the normal population, although cardiovascular and respiratory conditions and infections more common. Other conditions that contribute to mortality include extra-articular RA, especially pulmonary fibrosis [86], other complications of RA, and drug therapies. In the main, NSAIDs and corticosteroids have been implicated, and deaths directly due to DMARDS are reported to be low [86,91].

In recent years considerable attention has been drawn to the increase in cardiac mortality in RA because the inflammatory process itself may play an important role in the development of ischemic heart disease (IHD). The C-reactive protein and other inflammatory markers have been identified as independent risk factors for IHD [92] and controlling inflammation may well reduce the risk of IHD, despite therapies that themselves may contribute to atherogenesis. There is a complicated relationship between inflammatory activity, disease severity, and drug therapies used in RA with death from cardiovascular causes, which is not fully understood [93,94]. Although results from observational studies vary [95,96], there is a real possibility that better disease control could influence this outcome.

Age, sex, and functional ability are the most consistent risk factors reported for mortality in these RA studies. Although other features including severity of RA, inflammatory markers, functional disability, socioeconomic status, extra-articular RA, comorbidities, and RF have been associated with mortality, they have very variable prognostic importance. However, this is an important area because it raises the possibility of interventions to reduce mortality in RA [56]. RA may worsen or hasten a comorbidity, as Pincus and Callahan [97] claim for IHD, and these studies highlight the need in the rheumatology clinic to treat RA patients with active disease early and effectively [98] and to identify patients at additional risk from coexistent conditions and treat them actively or with preventative measures accordingly. This applies especially to cardiovascular comorbidity [99] and extra-articular RA (Box 7).

Extra-articular rheumatoid arthritis

Fortunately extra-articular features of RA are not common in early RA, and there is a clinical impression that these features are less common than 30–40 years ago. Nodules and Sjögren's syndrome remain the most common, reported in 10% and 4% at presentation and 29% and 7% by 5 years, respectively [58]. Other extra-articular features were all around 2% or less by 5 years. Nodules are associated with worse outcomes in RA, especially radiologic erosions and

---

Box 7. Mortality

- Modest increase in mortality in early RA
- Cardiovascular disease as main cause
- NSAIDs/COX2 have been implicated, but DMARDs rarely
- Predicted by age, sex, disease severity, and HAQ

---

mortality, but as they are not common early on, they do not feature much in prognostic indices [14].

Disease activity

Most early RA studies have shown an initial improvement in the majority of clinical and laboratory measures of disease activity and functional assessments when assessed from baseline for a year or two, and clinical trials report the same after initiation of drug therapy. The Middlesex and Bath cohorts were the first to report a subgroup of patients who continue to have very mild disease and even remission within 3 years, some as a result of second line medication but not all [17,18,67]. Subsequent inception cohorts have reported similar findings, although the frequency varies and this is partly due to differences in selection (population or community studies have milder RA at entry) but also the variation in the diagnostic criteria for clinical remission in RA. In general, around 10% to 20% of patients in inception cohorts achieve clinical remission [17,18,67, 100,101]. However, despite this a recent prospective study reported radiologic progression during a state of persistent remission [102].

Summary

The inception cohort approach has demonstrated a broader spectrum of disease course and outcome than the more numerous and larger longitudinal and retrospective studies. The latter have generally been in secondary or tertiary care and have thus selected the more severe and hospitalized RA patients, whereas some of the former have been primary care and community based, and milder disease. This factor is likely to explain some of the wide variations between studies described, identified in an editorial by Pincus and Callahan [103]. This may also explain the apparent loss of predictive power of some risk factors. The clinician needs to have reliable predictive markers both very early on and for the full spectrum of disease to guide decisions on drug therapies. It is at precisely this stage that the greatest fluctuations in clinical assessments occur, both at an individual level and with aggregated data. Prediction has undoubtedly improved from generally no better than 70% in previous decades to 90% in some recent studies. Some studies have shown that this has been achieved only by taking

---

Box 8. Summary

- Well designed inception cohorts provide invaluable information on medium- to long-term outcomes in RA
- Results reflect outcomes as a result of management practices for the specific population studied, but can be of general use
- Figures now available on work disability and need for orthopedic interventions are likely to be useful to patients and health service planners
- Prognostic factors vary in value according to outcome being measured
- Although reliability of prognostic factors has improved, clinical utility has yet to be confirmed and needs to be addressed
- Several cohorts have now been established worldwide that will provide data according to variations in treatment policies now and in the future

---

variables at 1 year [39,59,71], but this is still valuable information for clinicians. The problem arises in the move from predicting outcomes for groups of RA patients to forecasting the individual patient's likely course. Present evidence suggests a cautious approach and the rheumatologist needs to adjust current knowledge to the assessment of individual clinical presentations. The initiation of many inception cohorts has paralleled the development of early synovitis clinics and the earlier referral and earlier more aggressive interventions for RA [104], all of which are likely to improve long-term outcomes. Further inception cohorts have been set up in several countries in the last few years, often linked to national registers of RA, and this is likely to provide valuable contemporary information in an ever changing field (Box 8).

References

[1] Skekelle PG, Woolf SH, Eccles M, et al. The clinical guidelines: developing guidelines. BMJ 1999;318:593–6.
[2] Barton S. Which clinical studies provide best evidence? BMJ 2000;321:255–6.
[3] Choi HK, Seeger JD. Outcomes research in rheumatology. Rheumatic Clinics North Am 2004; 30(4):685–99.
[4] Van der Heide A, Jacobs JWG, Bijlsma JWJ, et al. The effectiveness of early treatment with second line antirheumatic drugs. Ann Intern Med 1996;124:699–707.
[5] Bird HA. Long-term safety monitoring in rheumatoid arthritis. A proposal from OMERACT. J Rheumatol 2000;37:831–3.
[6] Suarez-Almazor ME. In quest of the Holy Grail: efficacy versus effectiveness. J Rheumatol 2002;45:1–6.
[7] Furst DE. Observational Cohort Studies and Well Controlled Clinical Trials—we need them both. J Rheumatol 2004;31:1476–7.

[8] Felson D, Anderson J, Meenan R. The comparative efficacy and toxicity of second-line drugs in rheumatoid arthritis: results of two meta-analyses. Arthritis Rheum 1990;33:1449–61.

[9] Wolfe F, Hawley D, Cathey MA. Termination of slow acting anti rheumatic drugs in RA: a 14 year prospective evaluation of 1017 starts. J Rheumatol 1990;17:994–1002.

[10] Porter DR, McInnes I, Hunter J, et al. Outcome of second-line therapy in rheumatoid arthritis. Ann Rheum Dis 1995;53:812–5.

[11] Kremer JM. Rationale use of new and existing disease-modifying agents in rheumatoid arthritis. Ann Intern Med 2001;134:695–706.

[12] Smolen JS, Breedveld FC, Burmester GR, et al. Consensus statement on the initiation and continuation of tumour necrosis factor blocking therapies in rheumatoid arthritis. Ann Rheum Dis 2000;59:504–5.

[13] van der Heijde DMFM, van Reil PLCM, van de Putte LBA. Influence of prognostic features on final outcome in rheumatoid arthritis: a review of the literature. Semin Arthritis Rheum 1988; 17:284–92.

[14] Young A, van der Heijde DFM. Can we predict aggressive disease? Clin Rheumatol 1997;11:27–48.

[15] Kim JM, Weisman MH. When does rheumatoid arthritis begin and why do we need to know? Arthritis Rheum 2002;43:473–84.

[16] Wolfe F. Recommended reporting requirements for long-term observational studies in RA. J Rheumatol 1999;26:484–9.

[17] Fleming A, Crown JM, Corbett M. Prognostic value of early features in rheumatoid arthritis. BMJ 1976;i:1243–5.

[18] Jacoby RK, Jayson MI, Cosh JA. Onset, early stages, and prognosis of RA: a clinical study of 100 patients with 11 year follow up. BMJ 1973;2:96–100.

[19] Feigenbaum SL, Masi AT, Kaplan S. Prognosis in rheumatoid arthritis: a longitudinal study of newly diagnosed younger adult patients. Am J Med 1979;66:377–84.

[20] Fleming A, Crown J, Corbett M. Incidence of joint involvement in early rheumatoid arthritis. Rheumatol Rehabil 1976;15:92–6.

[21] Brooks A, Corbett M. Radiographic changes in early rheumatoid arthritis. Ann Rheum Dis 1977;36:71–3.

[22] Arnett FC, Edworthy SM, Bloch DA, et al. The ARA 1987 revised criteria for classification of rheumatoid arthritis. Arthritis Rheum 1988;31:315–24.

[23] Kellgren JH, Lawrence JS. Radiological assessment of rheumatoid arthritis. Ann Rheum Dis 1957;16:485–93.

[24] Larsen A, Dale K, Eek M. Radiographic evolution of rheumatoid arthritis and related conditions by standard reference films. Acta Radiol 1977;18:481–91.

[25] Sharp JT, Wolfe F, Mitchell DM. The progression of erosion and joint space narrowing scores in rheumatoid arthritis during the first twenty-five years of disease. Arthritis Rheum 1991; 34:660–7.

[26] Steinbrocker O, Traeger CH, Batterman RC. Therapeutic criteria in rheumatoid arthritis. JAMA 1949;140:659–62.

[27] Fries J, Spitz P, Young D. Dimensions of health outcomes: the health assessment questionnaire, disability and pain scales. J Rheumatol 1982;9:789–93.

[28] Ware J. Measuring patients' views: the optimum outcome measure. BMJ 1993;306:1429–30.

[29] van der Heijde DMFM, van T Hof MA, van Riel PLCM, et al. Judging disease activity in clinical practice in RA. First step in the development of a disease activity score. Ann Rheum Dis 1990;49:916–20.

[30] Felson DT, Anderson JJ, Boers M, et al. The American College of Rheumatology preliminary core set of disease activity measures for rheumatoid arthritis clinical trials. The committee on outcome measures in Rheumatoid Arthritis clinical trials. Arthritis Rheum 1993;36:729–40.

[31] Fex E, Jonsson K, Johnson U, Eberhardt K. Development of radiographic damage during the first 5–6 yr of RA: a prospective follow-up study of a Swedish cohort. Br J Rheumatol 1996; 35:1106–15.

[32] van der Heijde DMFM, van Riel PLCM, van Leeuwen MA, et al. Prognostic factors for radiographic damage and physical disability in early rheumatoid arthritis. Br J Rheumatol 1992; 8:519–26.

[33] van der Heijde DMFM, van Leeuwen A, van Riel PLCM, et al. Biannual radiographic assessments of hands and feet in a three-year prospective follow-up of patients with early rheumatoid arthritis. Arthritis Rheum 1992;35:26–33.

[34] van Zeben D, Hazes J, Zwinderman A, et al. Factors predicting outcome of rheumatoid arthritis: results of a follow-up study. J Rheumatol 1993;20:1288–96.

[35] Dixey J, Solymossy C, Jones P, et al. Structural damage as measured by radiographs accelerates between years two and three in early rheumatoid arthritis. Rheumatol 2004;43(Suppl. 2):344.

[36] Brennan P, Harrison B, Barrett E, et al. A simple algorithm to predict the development of radiological erosions in patients with early rheumatoid arthritis: prospective cohort study. BMJ 1996;313:471–6.

[37] Wolfe F, Sharp JT. Radiographic outcome of recent-onset RA: a 19-year study of radiographic progression. Arthritis Rheum 1998;41:1571–82.

[38] Graudal NA, Jurik AG, de Carvalho A, et al. Radiographic progression in RA: a long-term prospective study of 109 patients. Arthritis Rheum 1998;41(8):1470–80.

[39] Dixey J, Solymossy C, Young A. Is it possible to predict radiological damage in early RA? A report on occurrence, progression and prognostic factors for radiological erosions over first 3 years in 860 patients from early RA study (ERAS). J Rheumatol 2004;31(Suppl 69):48–54.

[40] Keen HI, Emery P. How should we manage early rheumatoid arthritis? From imaging to intervention. Curr Opin Rheumatol 2005;17:280–5.

[41] Kuper HH, van Leeuwen MA, van Riel PLCM, et al. Radiographic damage in large joints in early rheumatoid arthritis: relationship with radiographic damage in hands and feet, disease activity, and physical disability. Br J Rheumatol 1997;36:855–60.

[42] Winfield J, Cooke D, Brook A, et al. A prospective study of the radiological changes in the cervical spine in early rheumatoid arthritis. Ann Rheum Dis 1981;40:109–14.

[43] Winfield J, Young A, Williams P, et al. A prospective study of the radiological changes of hands, feet and cervical spine in adult rheumatoid disease. Ann Rheum Dis 1983;42:613–8.

[44] Young A, Corbett M, Winfield J, et al. A prognostic index for erosive changes in the hands, feet, and cervical spines in early rheumatoid arthritis. Br J Rheumatol 1988;27:94–101.

[45] Weyand CM, Hicok KC, Conn D, et al. The influence of HLA-DRB1 genes on disease severity in rheumatoid arthritis. J Clin Invest 1995;95:2120–6.

[46] Combe B, Dougados M, Goupile P, et al. Prognostic factors for radiographic damage in early rheumatoid arthritis. Arthritis Rheum 2000;44:1736–43.

[47] Mottonen T, Paimela L, Leirisalo-Repo M, et al. Only high disease activity and positive rheumatoid factor indicate poor prognosis in patients with early rheumatoid arthritis. Ann Rheum Dis 1998;57:533–9.

[48] Belghomari H, Saraux A, Allain J, et al. Risk factors for radiographic articular destruction of hands and wrists in rheumatoid arthritis. J Rheumatol 1999;26:2534–8.

[49] Harrison B, Thomson W, Symmons D, et al. The influence of HLA-DRB1 alleles and rheumatoid factor on disease outcome in an inception cohort of patients with early inflammatory arthritis. Arthritis Rheum 1999;42:2174–83.

[50] Bas S, Genevay S, Meyer O, et al. Anti-cyclic citrullinated peptide antibodies, IgM and IgA rheumatoid factors, in the diagnosis and prognosis of rheumatoid arthritis. Rheumatology (Oxford) 2003;42:677–80.

[51] Liang M, Larson M, Cullen K, et al. Comparative measurement efficiency and sensitivity of five health status instruments for arthritis research. Arthritis Rheum 1985;28:542–7.

[52] Fitzpatrick R, Ziebland S, Jenkinson C, et al. Importance of sensitivity to change as a criterion for selecting health status measures. Qual Health Care 1992;1:89–93.

[53] Fries JF. New instruments for assessing disability: not quite ready for prime time. Arthritis Rheum 2004;50:3064–7.

[54] Young A, Dixey J, Kulinskaya K, et al. Which patients stop working because of rheumatoid

arthritis? Results of five years' follow up in 732 patients from ERAS. Ann Rheum Dis 2002; 61:335–40.

[55] de Croon EM, Sluiter JK, Nijssen TF, et al. Predictive factors of work disability in rheumatoid arthritis: a systematic literature review. Ann Rheum Dis 2004;63:1362–7.

[56] Pincus T, Brooks RA, Callahan LF. Prediction of long-term mortality in patients with rheumatoid arthritis according to simple questionnaire and joint count measures. Ann Intern Med 1994;120:26–34.

[57] Eberhardt KB, Fex E. Functional impairment and disability in early rheumatoid arthritis— development over 5 years. J Rheumatol 1995;22:1037–42.

[58] Young A, Dixey J, Cox N, et al. How does functional disability in early rheumatoid arthritis affect patients and their lives? Results of 5yr follow up in 781 patients from the Early RA Study (ERAS). Rheumatology (Oxford) 2000;39:603–11.

[59] Wiles NJ, Dunn G, Barrett EM, et al. One year follow up variables predict disability 5 years after presentation with inflammatory polyarthritis with greater accuracy than at baseline. J Rheumatol 2000;27:2360–6.

[60] Combe B, Cantagrel A, Goupille P, et al. Predictive factors of 5-year health assessment questionnaire disability in early rheumatoid arthritis. J Rheumatol 2003;30:2344–9.

[61] Young A, Wilkinson P, Talamo J, et al. Socio-economic factors in the presentation and outcome of early rheumatoid arthritis. Lessons for the health service? Ann Rheum Dis 2000;59:794–9.

[62] van der Heide A, Jacobs JWG, Haanen HCM, et al. Is it possible to predict the first year extent of pain and disability for patients with rheumatoid arthritis? J Rheumatol 1995;22:1466–70.

[63] Matthews JNS, Altman DG, Campbell MJ, et al. Analysis of serial measurements in medical research. BMJ 1990;300:230–5.

[64] Hassell AB, Davis PD, Fowler PD, et al. Relationship between serial measures of disease activity and outcome in rheumatoid arthritis. Q J Med 1993;86:601–7.

[65] Carr A, Thompson P, Young A. Do health status measures (HSM) have a role in rheumatology? A survey of the use of and attitudes towards health status measures in the UK. Arthritis Rheum 1996;39:S261.

[66] Mitchell JM, Burkhauser RV, Pincus T. The importance of age, education, and comorbidity in the substantial earnings losses of individuals with symmetric polyarthritis. Arthritis Rheum 1988;31:348–57.

[67] Young A, Bielawska C, Corbett M, et al. A prospective study of early onset rheumatoid arthritis over fifteen years: prognostic features and outcome. Clin Rheumatol 1987;6(Suppl. 2):12–9.

[68] Fex E, Larsson B-M, Nived K, et al. Effect of RA on work status and social and leisure time activities in patients followed 8 years from onset. J Rheumatol 1998;25:44–50.

[69] Mau W, Bornmann M, Weber H, et al. Prediction of permanent work disability in a follow-up study of early rheumatoid arthritis: results of a tree structured analysis using recpam. Br J Rheumatol 1996;35:652–9.

[70] Barrett EM, Scott DGI, Wiles NJ, et al. The impact of rheumatoid arthritis on employment status in the early years of disease: a UK community-based study. Rheumatology (Oxford) 2000;39:1403–9.

[71] James D, Young A, Kulinskaya E, et al. Orthopaedic intervention in early rheumatoid arthritis. Occurrence and predictive factors in an inception cohort of 1029 patients followed for 5 years. Rheumatology (Oxford) 2004;43:369–76.

[72] Eberhardt KB, Fex E, Johnson U, et al. Association of HLA-DRB and DQB genes with two and five year outcome in rheumatoid arthritis. Ann Rheum Dis 1996;55:34–9.

[73] Wolfe F, Zwillich S. The long-term outcomes of rheumatoid arthritis. Arthritis Rheum 1998; 41:1072–82.

[74] Crilly A, Maiden N, Capell HA, Madhok R. Genotyping for disease associated HLA-DRβ1 alleles and the need for early joint surgery in rheumatoid arthritis: a quantitative evaluation. Ann Rheum Dis 1999;58:114–7.

[75] Hakala M, Nieminen P, Koivisto O. More evidence from a community based series of better outcome in rheumatoid arthritis. J Rheumatol 1994;21:1432–7.

[76] Gossec L, Bettembourg-Brault I, Pham T, et al. HLA DRB1*01 and DRB1*04 phenotyping does not predict the need for joint surgery in rheumatoid arthritis. A retrospective quantitative evaluation of 300 French patients. Clin Exp Rheumatol 2004;22:462–4.

[77] Van Jaarsveld CH, Otten HG, Jacobs JW, et al. Association of HLA-DR with susceptibility to and expression of rheumatoid arthritis: re-evaluation by means of genomic tissue typing. Br J Rheumatol 1998;38:411–6.

[78] Symmons DPM. Mortality in rheumatoid arthritis. Br J Rheumatol 1988;44(Suppl 1):44–54.

[79] Wolfe F, Mitchell DM, Sibley PW, et al. The mortality of rheumatoid arthritis. Arthritis Rheum 1994;37:481–94.

[80] Gabriel SE, Crowson CS, Kremers HM, et al. Survival in rheumatoid arthritis. Arthritis Rheum 2003;48:54–8.

[81] Prior P, Symmons DPM, Scott DL, et al. Cause of death in rheumatoid arthritis. Br J Rheumatol 1984;23:92–9.

[82] Riise T, Jacobsen BK, Gran JT, et al. Total mortality is increased in rheumatoid arthritis. A 17-year prospective study. Clin Rheumatol 2001;20:123–7.

[83] Corbett M, Young A, Dalton D, et al. Factors predicting death, survival and functional outcome in a prospective study of early rheumatoid disease over fifteen years. Br J Rheumatol 1993;32:717–23.

[84] Lindqvist E, Eberhardt K. Mortality in rheumatoid arthritis patients with disease in the 1980s. Ann Rheum Dis 1999;58:11–4.

[85] Kroot EJA, van Leuuwen MA, van Rijswijk MH, et al. No increased mortality in patients with rheumatoid arthritis: up to 10 years follow-up from disease onset. Ann Rheum Dis 2000;59:954–8.

[86] Mattey D, Thompson W, Ollier W, et al. Association of the HLA-DRB1 shared epitope with mortality in rheumatoid arthritis. Arthritis Rheum 2004;50(Suppl):1280.

[87] Reilly P, Cosh JA, Maddison PJ, et al. Mortality and survival in rheumatoid arthritis: a 25-year study of 100 patients. Ann Rheum Dis 1990;49:363–9.

[88] Goodson NJ, Wiles NJ, Lunt M, et al. Mortality in early inflammatory polyarthritis. Arthritis Rheum 2002;46(8):2010–9.

[89] Mikuls TR, Saag KG, Criswell LA, et al. Mortality risk associated with rheumatoid arthritis in a prospective cohort of older women: results from the IOWA Women's Health Study. Ann Rheum Dis 2002;61:994–9.

[90] Ward M. Recent improvements in survival in patients with rheumatoid arthritis: better outcomes or different study designs? Arthritis Rheum 2001;44:1467–9.

[91] Myllykangas-Luosujarvi R, Aho K, Isomaki H. Death attributed to antirheumatic medication in a nationwide series of 1666 patients with rheumatoid arthritis who have died. J Rheumatol 1995;22:2200–2.

[92] Ridker P, Cushman M, Stampfer M, et al. Inflammation, aspirin and the risk of cardiovascular disease in apparently healthy men. N Engl J Med 1997;336(14):973–9.

[93] Bacon PA, Townsend JN. Nails in the coffin: increasing evidence for the role of rheumatic disease in the cardiovascular mortality of rheumatoid arthritis. Arthritis Rheum 2001;44:2707–10.

[94] Kitas GD, Erb N. Tackling ischaemic heart disease in rheumatoid arthritis. Rheumatology (Oxford) 2003;42:607–13.

[95] Galindo-Rodriguez G, Avira Zubrieta J, Russell A, et al. Disappointing long term results with disease modifying anti rheumatic drugs. A practice based study. J Rheumatol 1999;16:237–43.

[96] Krause D, Schleusser B, Herborn G, et al. Response to methotrexate treatment is associated with reduced mortality in patients with severe rheumatoid arthritis. Arthritis Rheum 2000;43:14–21.

[97] Pincus T, Callahan L. Taking mortality in rheumatoid arthritis seriously – predictive markers, socioeconomic status and comorbidity. J Rheumatol 1986;13:841–5.

[98] Pincus T, Gibofsky A, Weinblatt ME. Urgent care and tighter control of rheumatoid arthritis as in diabetes and hypertension: better treatments but a shortage of rheumatologists. Arthritis Rheum 2002;46:851–4.

[99] Boers M, Dijkmans B, Gabriel S, et al. Making an impact on mortality in rheumatoid arthritis. Arthritis Rheum 2004;50:1734–9.

[100] Eberhardt K, Fex E. Clinical course and remission rate in patients with early rheumatoid arthritis: relationship to outcome after five years. Br J Rheumatol 1998;37:1324–9.

[101] Prevoo ML, van Gestel AM, van't Hof MA, et al. Remission in a prospective study of rheumatoid arthritis. American Rheumatism Association preliminary remission criteria in relation to the disease activity score. Br J Rheumatol 1996;35:1101–5.

[102] Molenar ETH, Voskuyl AE, Dinant HJ, et al. Progression of radiologic damage in patients with rheumatoid arthritis in clinical remission. Arthritis Rheum 2004;50:36–42.

[103] Pincus T, Callahan LF. Prognostic markers of activity and damage in rheumatoid arthritis: why trials and inception cohort studies indicate more favourable outcomes than studies with more established disease. Br J Rheumatol 1995;34:196–9.

[104] Emery P. Therapeutic approaches for early rheumatoid arthritis. How early? How aggressive? Br J Rheumatol 1995;34(Suppl 2):87–90.

[105] Kaarela K. Prognostic factors and diagnostic criteria in early rheumatoid arthritis. Scand J Rheumatol 1985;57:1–54.

[106] Isomaki H, Martio J, Sarna S, et al. Predicting outcome of rheumatoid arthritis. A Soviet-Finnish cooperative study. Scand J Rheumatol 1984;13:33–8.

[107] Berlin Collaborating Rheumatology Study Group. HLA-DRB1 genes, rheumatoid factor, elevated C-reactive protein: independent risk factors in early rheumatoid arthritis. J Rheumatol 2000;27:2100–9.

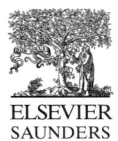

RHEUMATIC
DISEASE CLINICS
OF NORTH AMERICA

Rheum Dis Clin N Am 31 (2005) 681–698

Conventional X-Ray in Early Arthritis

Annelies Boonen, MD, PhD*,
Désirée van der Heijde, MD, PhD

*Division of Rheumatology, Department of Internal Medicine, University Hospital Maastricht Care and
Public Health Research Institute, University Maastricht, Maastricht, The Netherlands*

The importance of early identification of patients with inflammatory arthritis and in particular identifying patients at risk of an unfavorable long-term outcome is recognized. Patients who develop a persistent or erosive arthritis are considered to have an unfavorable long-term outcome. Rheumatoid arthritis (RA), oligoarthritis, polyarticular psoriatic arthritis (PsA), and the other spondyloarthropathies (SpAs) all are inflammatory conditions that place patients at risk of developing persistent or erosive disease. The role of conventional radiology of peripheral joints is well established for RA and has been studied increasingly for PsA, but less so for the other SpAs. This situation is due at least in part to primarily axial involvement in these conditions. In RA, radiographic damage can be assessed by several scoring systems. These methods have proved to be reliable and sensitive to changes that are clinically relevant. In addition, data from numerous clinical trials and cohort studies have shown that radiographic damage progresses linearly over time, reflects cumulative disease activity, is linked to functional outcome, and can be suppressed by disease controlling antirheumatic therapies (DCARTs).

In the preclassification stage of early inflammatory arthritis (EIA), the role of conventional radiology has not been explored fully with respect to the diagnostic or prognostic value or with respect to progression of damage. EIA differs from the classic diagnostic entities in many aspects. The spectrum of patients included is heterogeneous from a diagnostic and from a prognostic point of view. Patients can present with monarticular, oligoarticular, or polyarticular disease, and any

* Corresponding author. Division of Rheumatology, Department of Internal Medicine, University Hospital Maastricht and Care and Public Health Research Institute (CAPHRI), University Maastricht, P. Debyelaan 25, PO Box 5800, 6202 AZ, Maastricht, The Netherlands.
E-mail address: aboo@sint.azm.nl (A. Boonen).

joint site can be involved. Many patients have self-limiting arthritis, which is unlikely to become erosive, whereas a few patients develop severe destructive disease. This latter group of patients likely has no radiographic abnormalities at the first evaluation. When treated early, patients with erosive disease show less progression than observed in advanced disease and may show repair when treated with drugs able to induce repair. The data available on assessing radiographic damage in RA or PsA cannot simply be transferred to patients with EIA with respect to diagnosis, prognosis, or evaluation of progression. This article reviews the literature on conventional radiographic assessments of peripheral joints in cohorts of patients with EIA. Also, specific issues on conventional radiology in EIA compared with early RA and early PsA are discussed. Finally, the role of conventional radiography in EIA is considered.

Overview of cohorts reporting radiographic assessment in patients with early inflammatory arthritis

Conventional radiographs have been included as outcome measures in several EIA cohorts. Publications that limited the analyses of radiographic data to patients who fulfilled at inclusion criteria for RA [1,2] or PsA [3] are excluded in this overview because they represent early RA or early PsA. Table 1 presents the design of the six cohort studies with emphasis on the patient inclusion criteria, method to assess and report radiographic outcome, and results of the radiographic outcome.

Cohorts differed with respect to the maximum disease duration at inclusion and the definition of the diagnoses at the final follow-up. Radiographs of hands and feet were included in all cohorts, but methods to assess damage in hands and feet were not uniform. Further, the following specific characteristics of some studies should be considered when interpreting the results. In the Norfolk Arthritis Register (NOAR), radiographs were not systematically performed at inclusion [4,5]. In the Austria Early Arthritis (EA) Action, radiographic data are limited to patients fulfilling criteria of RA at 1-year follow-up [6]. In the Amsterdam EA Cohort, the patients with PsA at baseline were excluded, and radiologic data were presented only for the patients with undifferentiated arthritis (UA) or RA at inclusion [7]. In addition to the radiographs of hands and feet, symptomatic large joints were imaged in the Austrian EA Action [6] and the sacroiliac joints were imaged in the Brittany EA Cohort [8,9], but findings of these films were not yet reported.

Baseline radiographic findings of hands and feet in early inflammatory arthritis and baseline damage as predictor of final diagnosis

In the Brittany EA Cohort, 15% of patients had erosions in their hands or feet at baseline ($n = 149$), 32.5% in the group that was classified at the 2 years as RA

(37%) compared with 5.5% of patients classified at 2 years as non-RA ($P < .02$) [8,9]. Baseline Sharp scores in the hands ($n = 285$) were 5.9 and 2.5 in the RA and non-RA groups ($P < .001$) and in the feet ($n = 149$) were 2.3 and 1.2 in the RA and non-RA groups. The authors studied the radiographic item of the American College of Rheumatology (ACR) 1987 criteria for RA (item 7). This item considers erosions or decalcification in the joints of fingers or wrists. Sensitivity and specificity of this radiographic criterion in patients with EIA, to predict the expert's diagnosis of RA at 2 years, was reported first when using the radiographs of hands only. The results were compared with sensitivity and specificity after including the radiographs of the feet and when applying the full Sharp score instead of erosions and decalcification only. First, it was concluded that decalcification had a low reliability. The addition of assessing erosions of the feet improved sensitivity (from 17% to 33%), while maintaining specificity (95%). Quantification of erosions and including joint space narrowing by applying the Sharp score modified by Plant did not improve test characteristics [10]. The positive and negative predictive values of erosions in hands and feet in this population were 75% (positive predictive value) and 29% (negative predictive value).

In the Leiden EA Cohort, 15% of all patients were erosive at baseline [11]. In the predictive model for unfavorable outcome, the authors used a prognostic classification instead of the classic classifications and distinguished persistent synovitis (16%) and erosive disease (24%) as the unfavorable outcomes as opposed to self-limiting disease (60%) after 1 year. They showed that erosions at baseline predicted persistent synovitis (relative risk 2.75) and progressive erosive disease (relative risk infinite) after 2 years. Other predictors of erosive disease (compared with nonerosive persistence) were morning stiffness lasting longer than 1 hour, arthritis in more than three joint groups, bilateral compression pain in the metatarsophalangeal joints, presence of rheumatoid factor (RF), and presence of anticitrulline peptide.

In the Amsterdam EA Cohort, patients with RA meeting the 1987 ACR criteria were distinguished at inclusion from patients with undifferentiated oligoarthritis or undifferentiated polyarthritis (UPA) [7]. After 1-year follow-up, the latter group was classified as mild or progressive UPA, based on either a Sharp score greater than or equal to 10 points, increase of radiographic damage 4 or more Sharp points, or a Health Assessment Questionnaire (HAQ) score greater than or equal to 1. Total Sharp scores, but not frequency of erosive disease, were reported. In patients with the final diagnosis of mild UA, the median Sharp score at baseline was 2 (range 0–55) compared with 8 (range 0–58) and 5 (range 0–136) in patients classified at follow-up as progressive UPA or RA.

Of the National Institutes of Health Early Synovitis (ES) Cohort, 8% was erosive at baseline, with 18% of patients classified as having RA and 5% of patients classified as having non-RA ($P < .01$) erosions at follow-up. In a subgroup of 66 patients, serum matrix metalloproteinase-1 (MMP-1) and C-reactive protein (CRP) differed between erosive and nonerosive patients ($P < .01$). Proteinases did not discriminate RA from non-RA [12,13].

Table 1
Overview of studies reporting outcome of conventional radiographs in patients with early inflammatory arthritis

Cohort (start year), first author, year [Ref.]	Inclusion, exclusion, and clinical outcome[a]	Radiographic characteristics	Radiographic outcome reported	Patients in whom radiography reported	Radiographic outcome	Comments
NIH ES Cohort (1994), Goldbach-Mansky, 2000 [12]; Goldbach-Mansky, 2000 [13]	*Inclusion:* synovitis ≥ 1 joint, ≥ 6 wk, < 12 mo. *Exclusion:* septic arthritis, crystal arthritis, defined systemic disease. *Clinical outcome:* RA diagnosis at 1 y according to ACR 1987 criteria.	Hands and feet at baseline and at 12 mo. Erosion: definite loss of cortical lining in ≥ 2 joints. Radiologists blinded for patient characteristics.	Definite erosion at baseline. Cross-sectional association between serum MMPs and TIMPs and erosive disease.	238 patients. *At 1 y:* 45% RA; 9% ReA; 6% PsA or other SpA; 5% other; 35% UA. 96% of patients in RA group at 1 y had RA at inclusion [12]. 66/238 patients had synovial tissue samples and serum assessments of MMP and TMP proteinases [13].	*Baseline:* 18% in RA group at follow-up and 5% in the non-RA group were erosive (P < 0.01). *At 1 y:* 36% in RA group. *Association erosions MMP:* MMP-1 in serum associated with erosions (yes/no) but NOT with the distinction RA and non-RA [13].	Results of paired films were only reported in patients with early RA and not included in this review.
Brittany EA Cohort, (1995–1997 GP referral) Devauchelle-Pensec, 2001 [8]; Devauchelle-Pensec 2004 [9]	*Inclusion:* < 1 y synovitis; ≥ 16-y-old; ≥ 1 swollen joint; no previous diagnosis other arthritis. *Evaluation stopped:* if clinical diagnosis of defined joint disease and fulfils published	Hands at baseline and biannually thereafter. Pelvic radiograph at baseline. Erosions, decalcification, or both in hands (item 7 of ACR criteria RA) and/or feet. Sharp score of hands	Reliability of scoring erosions and/or decalcification in the hands (item 7 of ACR criteria RA) and/or feet (n = 130 films). Agreement between blinded observer and unblinded office	258/270 patients for assessment including hand radiography only [8] and 149/270 patient in study on feet and hand radiography [9]. At last visit (mean follow-up of 30 mo) 36%	*Baseline:* Erosions: hands: 17% of RA and 4% of non-RA (P < 0.001); feet: 18% of RA and 2% non-RA (P < 0.02). Decalcification: hands: 5.5% of RA	

criteria of joint disease. *Clinical outcome:* expert panel classification of RA or non-RA, based on clinical, laboratory and radiologic features after final visit (mean follow-up 30 mo). Sensitivity and specificity of ACR 1987 criteria for expert diagnosis (91% and 75%).

and Plant modification of Sharp for the feet: erosion, narrowing and total score. 1 observer blind for patient characteristics. Intraobserver (6 mo) and interobserver variability on subset of 130 films.

based rheumatologist on erosions and decalcification in hands (item 7 ACR criteria). Comparative sensitivity and specificity for RA at follow-up; erosions, and/or decalcification in hands and/or feet; Sharp score of hands and/or hands and feet combined (best cut-off based on receiver operator curves).

of patients had expert diagnosis of RA.

and 8.5% of non-RA; feet: 3.5% of RA and 4% of non-RA. Sharp score: hands: 5.9 in RA and 2.5 in non-RA ($P < 0.001$); feet: 2.3 in RA and 1.2 in non-RA ($P < 0.004$). *Reliability:* Intraobserver variation; erosions: hands: 0.88; feet: 0.87. Decalcification: hands: 0.65; feet: 0.52 Interobserver variation Sharp: hands: 0.98; feet: 0.90; agreement for item 7 hands rheumatologist/ observer: 0.29. *Sensitivity and specificity for clinical diagnosis RA:* Erosions: hands: 17% and 96%;

(continued on next page)

Table 1 (*continued*)

Cohort (start year), first author, year [Ref.]	Inclusion, exclusion, and clinical outcome[a]	Radiographic characteristics	Radiographic outcome reported	Patients in whom radiography reported	Radiographic outcome	Comments
Brittany EA Cohort, (1995–1997 GP referral) Devauchelle-Pensec, 2001 [8]; Devauchelle-Pensec 2004 [9]					feet: 18% and 98%; hands and feet: 33% and 95%. Sharp erosion score: hands and feet: (cutoff 3.5) 28% and 90%.	
NOAR (1990–1994 GP referral), Bukhari, 2001 [5]; Bukhari, 2002 [4]	*Inclusion:* ≥ 6 y or; ≥ 2 swollen joint; ≥ 4 wk; new referrals (most < 3 y). *Excluded:* other than UPA, RA, postviral arthritis, PsA. *Clinical outcome:* diagnosis RA according to ACR 1987 criteria.	Hands and feet: (1) Within 24 mo if 3 ACR criteria at first follow-up visit or if classification RA could be made in case erosion would be detected. (2) All patients at y 5 (mean time interval 48 mo). Larsen method: Erosive: score ≥ 2 in individual joint 2 or 3 readers blind for sequence. Consensus if discrepancy. Intraobserver and interobserver agreement 90% and 81%.	Erosive in function of symptom duration [5]. Predictors of progression in those with paired films [4].	416/759 patients contributed films for analyses of first occurrence of erosions [5]. 439 patients contributed to study of paired films. By 5 y 75% had RA [4].	*Study first erosion [5]:* Of 337 patients with a first film within 24 mo (suspected RA), 36% erosive. In those not erosive or suspected of RA after 24 mo, 23%, 28% and 47% became erosive in the 2nd, 3rd, and 4th year [5]. *Study paired films [4]:* 33% erosive at first film (median symptom duration 24 mo) and 49% at second film;	Films were not systematically taken at baseline.

Leiden EA Clinic (1993 GP referral and regular rheumatology clinic), Visser, 2002 [11]	*Inclusion:* ≥ 1 swollen joint; ≤ 2 y symptoms; first contact with a rheumatologist. *Follow-up stops:* after 1 y: if transient synovitis OR in remission in case the diagnosis was crystal synovitis or trauma or reactive arthritis, sarcoid arthritis or UA. *Clinical outcome:* self-limited arthritis (or remission), persis-	Hands and feet at inclusion, 6 mo and yearly afterwards. Chest radiograph. SHS method: erosive: erosion score ≥ 1 1 reader blinded for patient characteristics (not stated if chronologic).	Erosive arthritis compared to persistent nonerosive or self-limited arthritis. Erosion(s) as predictor of persistent and erosive disease.	524/566 patients in the follow up at 2 y *At follow-up:* 30% RA, 26% UA, 11% crystal-induced arthritis, 6% OA, 5% sarcoid, 15% other (including PsA); 60% self-limiting, 16% persistent nonerosive. and 24% persistent erosive.	increase of Larsen from mean of 2 to 7 over a mean of 48 mo; Larsen first film associated with baseline CRP (highest tertile) and RF; Larsen last film mainly predicted by Larsen baseline and to lesser extent CRP and RF. *Baseline:* Erosive: 15%. *At 2 y:* Erosive: 24%. (of those 83% RA, 6% UA, 5% PsA, 1.6% SpA. *Erosions as predictor of outcome:* Predicts (1) persistent synovitis [OR 2.75] and (2). erosive disease [OR infinite].

(continued on next page)

Table 1 (*continued*)

Cohort (start year), first author, year [Ref.]	Inclusion, exclusion, and clinical outcome[a]	Radiographic characteristics	Radiographic outcome reported	Patients in whom radiography reported	Radiographic outcome	Comments
Leiden EA Clinic (1993 GP referral and regular rheumatology clinic), Visser, 2002 [11]	tent synovitis or erosive after (1 or) 2 y; remission: 6 mo symptom-free and no DMARD. *Other classifications:* ACR 1987 criteria RA.					
Austrian EA Action (1995), Machold, 2002 [6]	*Inclusion:* ≤ 12 wk; swelling in ≥ 1 joint without trauma; pain in ≥ 1 joint with morning stiffness > 60 min. *At least 1 lab:* RF+, ESR > 20, CR P > 5, leucocytes > upper limit normal. *Clinical outcome:* 1958 ACR criteria RA.	Hands and feet at entry and yearly afterwards. Other involved joints if applicable. Larsen method: Erosive: score ≥2 in at least one joint; Total score. 2 rheumatologists and 2 radiologists in one session. Blind for chronology. Test-retest: 0.86.	Erosive at baseline and 1 y. Soft tissue swelling at baseline. Score: mean (SD).	108/219 had at least 1-y follow-up. 66 of those had final diagnosis RA at y 1. *At 1 y:* 61% RA, 13% UA, 2% PsA. Radiographic outcome reported in those with final diagnosis RA (n = 66).	*Of RA patients:* *Erosive:* baseline: 12%; 1 y: 28%; *Soft tissue swelling:* baseline: 21%. *Larsen score:* baseline: 3.5 (6.6); 1 y: 6.3 (10.9). *Predictors of becoming erosive:* RF [OR: 9.7(1.05–89.93)].	No radiographic data on patients who had no final diagnosis RA.

| Amsterdam EA Clinic (1995–1998), Jansen, 2000 [7] | Inclusion: > 18 y; ≥ 2 joints; < 3 y. Exclusion: previous DMARD; diagnosis of ReA, PsA, crystal arthritis, OA, sarcoidosis, bacterial arthritis, defined systemic disease. Clinical outcome: 1987 ACR criteria for RA for those already fulfilling thse criteria at entry; if at baseline UPA, the 1-y follow-up considered arthritis [1] progressive; if radiographic progression ≥ 4 points, radiographic score ≥ 10 or HAQ ≥ 1 or [2] mild; if not progressive. | Hands and feet at baseline and 1 y. SHS method: Total Sharp score. 1 observer blind for patient characteristics and chronology. | Predictors for progressive UPA at 1 y. Predictors for radiographic damage/progression in the entire group at 1 y. | 323 patients eligible, 316 could be contacted and 280 participated. At baseline: 72% RA; 27% UA (58% polyarthritis and 24% oligoarthritis). At y 1: 58% (n = 45) mild UPA and 42% progressive (n = 32) of which 10 fulfilled ACR criteria for RA. | Baseline median Sharp: Mild UPA: 2.0 Progressive UPA: 0.9 RA: 1.1 1-y mean Sharp: Mild UPA: 2.0 Progressive UPA: 12.5 RA: 9.5. 1-y mean Sharp progression: Mild UPA: 0 Progressive UPA: 3.0 (it was mentioned there was no difference between RA and non-RA) RA: 4.5. Predictors progressive UPA: Age [OR:1.5], arthritis hands [OR: 4.2] (uncertain if radiographic score at baseline was included in analysis). | Patients excluded if not classified after 1 y into progressive and not progressive. The progressive UPA were not separately analysed for RA or non-RA, but it was mentioned that progressive UPA diagnosed as RA were not different from other progressive UPA patients with regard to radiographic progression. |

Abbreviations: NIH, National Institutes of Health; OA, osteoarthritis; TIMPs, tissue inhibitors of metalloproteinases.

a Description outcome at follow-up.

Progression and predictors of radiographic damage over time

NOAR suggests that the proportion of patients with EIA who become erosive is linear. In patients classified as having RA or suspected to have RA in the first 24 months after inclusion, 36% were erosive at entry into the cohort. In patients not erosive on the first film, 23%, 38%, and 47% were erosive 2, 3, and 4 years after symptom onset [5]. In patients with paired films within the first 5 years, 33% were erosive at the first film, and 49% were erosive after a mean interval of 48 months [4]. During that period, the Larsen score progressed from 2 to 7 points. In the Leiden EA Cohort, the proportion of patients with erosive disease increased from 15% at inclusion to 24% after 2 years [11].

Within the Austrian EA Action, more substantial progression was seen, but the analyses were limited to patients classified as having RA at the 1-year follow-up (61% of all EIA) [6]. At baseline, 12% were erosive, increasing to 28% at follow-up. Of patients with RA at 1 year, 68% had RA at the baseline. RF at baseline predicted development of erosions during the first year.

In the Amsterdam EA Cohort, 42% of patients with UPA were classified as progressive at 1 year [7]. Mean progression in Sharp score was zero points in the mild UPA group, 3 in the progressive UPA group, and 3.5 in the initial RA group. In patients with progressive UPA, 31% fulfilled ACR 1987 criteria for RA at follow-up, but radiographic progression was not different in these patients compared with the non-RA patients in this group. Progressive UPA could be predicted by age (odds ratio [OR] 1.05) and presence of arthritis in the hands (OR 4.2). It is not clear if baseline Sharp scores were included in the multivariate regression. DCARTs were given in 86% of patients with a final diagnosis of progressive UPA and in 100% of patients with the initial diagnosis of RA.

Relationship between radiographic damage and functioning

The relationship between radiographic damage and functional outcome was not examined in any of the studies. In the Amsterdam EA Cohort, mean HAQ score improved approximately 0.2 in patients with mild UPA, showed no change in patients with progressive UPA, and improved by approximately 0.3 points in patients with the initial diagnosis of RA [7].

Issues in conventional radiology in early inflammatory arthritis and comparison with early rheumatoid arthritis and psoriatic arthritis

Diagnosis: joints, features, and scoring method

EIA is a descriptive and not a diagnostic concept. Conventional radiographs at the first presentation of a patient with EIA can help to make a classic diagnosis because the radiographs allow application of the established knowledge of that diagnosis to these patients. Up to now, all radiographic studies in EIA concentrated on the role of erosions or joint space narrowing in hands or feet and on the contribution to predict RA in an early stage. Erosions and joint space narrowing are not a unique feature of RA, however. In the French EA Cohort, erosions in hands and feet had a high (95%) specificity for the expert's diagnosis of RA, but the diagnostic considerations in patients with erosions but without RA were not discussed [8,9]. In the Leiden EA cohort, most (83.5%) patients with erosive disease after 2 years fulfilled the ACR 1987 classification for RA, but 5.5% had PsA, 1.6% had SpAs, and 6.3% had UA [11]. In the Amsterdam EA Cohort, radiographic progression in patients with progressive UPA was similar in patients classified as having RA compared with non-RA [7].

To improve classification (diagnosis) and to establish prognosis, it is important to consider features other than erosions and joint space narrowing, and sites other than those traditionally evaluated in RA should be assessed. In the French study, it was shown that decalcification (part of item 7, the radiographic criterion of the 1987 criteria for RA) as a separate feature had low reliability and was not explored further with regard to test characteristics [8]. The relevance of features such as periostitis and bone apposition and of imaging additional joints (eg, the distal interphalangeal joints or large joints) needs to be clarified, however. Rahman and colleagues [14] compared radiographic damage of 39 RA and 42 PsA patients who were matched for gender and age (within 10 years) and had a mean disease duration of 6.1 and 6.9 years, respectively. Conventional films of hands and feet were assessed for abnormalities by the Steinbrocker score modified for PsA (including distal interphalangeal joints of the hands and interphalangeal joints of the feet). In addition, several additional abnormal features were recorded. In the hands periostitis was observed in 2.6% of RA patients compared with 9.5% of PsA patients, and bony proliferation was observed in 2.6% of RA patients compared with 4.8% of PsA patients. Dactylitis was not seen in RA, but was seen in 7.1% of patients with PsA. None of these differences were significant, and for the feet the differences were even less pronounced. This was a study in patients with established disease. Three studies reported radiographic abnormalities in early PsA, but did not report on features other than erosions and narrowing and did not compare the additive value of including distal interphalangeal joints in the scores [3,15,16].

The diagnostic (or prognostic) value of including large joint radiographs in the initial assessment of a patient with EIA has not been studied. For RA, it is established that patients who are nonerosive in the hands and feet do not have erosions in large joints [17]. In the St. Vincent's Early PsA Cohort, the relevance of imaging of the sacroiliac joints was studied. At a median of 24 months (range 11–56), sacroiliitis was seen in 17% of patients (unilateral in 60%) [3].

Magnitude of structural damage and progression over time

Limited data are available to estimate the magnitude of progression of joint damage in patients with EIA. Considering the studies analyzing unselected EIA patients (ie, not limited to patients with the follow-up diagnosis of RA), 8% [13] to 15% [11,18] of patients had erosions in hands or feet at baseline. The progression of patients with erosive disease was reported only in the Leiden EA Cohort, which increased from 15% to 24% after 2 years [11]. Although in the analyses of NOAR, the clinician's suspicion of the ACR diagnosis of RA influenced the decision to obtain radiographic assessment, the results suggest a fairly linear increase in the number of patients becoming erosive over time (23% at 2 years, 28% at 3 years, and 47% at 4 years) [5]. Progression in radiographic scores was not reported for unselected patients with EIA. In the NOAR, the Larsen progression (range 0–190) was 5 points over a mean of 48 months (2.5 per year; 1.5% of the maximal score) [4]. In the Austrian EA Action, the progression in mean Larsen (range 0–160) over 1 year was 2.8 points (1.75% of the maximal score) [6]. In the Amsterdam study, mean progression of the Sharp score (range 0–448) was 3 over 1 year (0.67% of maximal score) in patients with progressive UPA compared with 4.5 in patients with RA (1% of maximal score) [7]. Of patients with UPA at baseline, 42% were progressive over the 1-year period. The magnitude of radiographic progression was similar in all patients with progressive UPA, independent of whether they fulfilled at the final visits 1987 ACR classification criteria for RA. The films of the NOAR, the Austrian EA Action, and the Amsterdam cohort were scored by readers blind for chronology. None of the studies reported on the presence of negative scores. The box plots of the radiographic change in Sharp score in the Amsterdam publication indicate a large proportion of negative scores.

Comparison between studies, and even more so between EIA, early RA, and early PsA, needs to be done with caution. Of patients in early RA cohorts, 5% [19] to 77% [20] had erosions at inclusion, and 80% of patients had erosions after 5 years [19]. The occurrence of erosions over time was linear, at least in the first years of the disease. Yearly progression in the Larsen score of hands and feet in three EIA cohorts was estimated to be 3.8 units per year (2.5% of possible damage) compared with 6 points per year in three studies that applied the Sharp score of hands and feet (1.3% of possible damage) [21]. In early RA, there is evidence that the radiographic damage and progression of damage has become less severe in recent years. Sokka and colleagues [22] compared radiographic outcome in three consecutive Finnish EA Cohorts (≤1 or 2 years). Cohort A included patients between 1983 and 1985, Cohort B included patients between 1988 and 1989, and Cohort C included patients between 1995 and 1996. Although the increase in patients with at least one erosion over 5 years was only slightly lower in the later cohorts, the decline in patients with important radiographic damage defined as Larsen score greater than 10 was significant. The proportions of patients with a Larsen score greater than 10 were 8.7%, 0%, and 2.6% at baseline and 54.5% (+45.8%), 32.6% (+32.6%), and 14% (+11.4) after 5 years in Cohorts A, B, and C. The median 5-year progression in Larsen score (0–100) in hands and feet was 12 (2.4 per year; 2.4% of maximal score), 6 (1.2 per year; 1.2% of maximal score), and 4 (0.8 per year; 0.8% of maximal score) over 5 years in Cohorts A, B, and C.

The more important influence on the cumulative radiographic damage compared with the proportion of patients having erosions illustrates that both outcomes have additional value, at least in early RA. For RA, a simplified scoring method (Simple Erosion and Narrowing Scale: SENS) was developed, including the same joints as in the Sharp van der Heijde Score (SHS) and counting the number of eroded joints and the number of narrowed joints (0–86). In early RA, this method showed similar sensitivity to change as the SHS [23]. Because the data in EIA suggest the increase in number of erosive patients was linear over time, this method might prove interesting in EIA. When evaluating progression, the time period wherein changes can be reliably detected is relevant. Bruynesteyn and colleagues [24] showed it was possible to detect changes reliably (higher than the smallest detectable change) by the SHS for RA after 3 months of follow-up, especially when scored in chronologic order. The likelihood of progression was higher in patients with established RA compared with early RA, influencing the sample sizes required for studies.

Data on progression of structural damage in early PsA are limited. In NOAR (early PsA with isolated axial disease excluded), 22% were erosive at baseline, and median Larsen score was 2.5 [15]. Punzi and colleagues [16] compared patients with young onset (≤ 60 years old) and elderly (> 60 years old) onset early (≤ 1 year) PsA. After 2 years, the mean number of erosions in the hands had increased from 2.4 to 4.4 in the younger group and from 2.2 to 2.7 in the older group of patients. In the feet, the number of erosions increased from 2.7 to 4.7 and from 1.1 to 2.1 in the younger and older groups. In the early PsA cohort of the St. Vincent ES clinic, 26% were erosive at baseline, and 47% were erosive after a median follow-up of 24 months (Sharp PsA method) [3]. The number of joints with erosions was highest in the hands at baseline, but in the feet at follow-up. In the latter group, the increase measured by the Sharp PsA method was 1.6 for erosions (0.8 per year; 0.3% of maximal damage) and 1.8 for narrowing (0.9 per year; 0.4% of maximal damage). An observation was made during a drug intervention trial with respect to the sensitivity to change of features considered specific for PsA (periostitis and tuft resorption) with respect to the influence of including the distal interphalangeal joints on the sensitivity to change of the Sharp score for PsA [25]. Although important differences were seen in the total Sharp PsA score between the treatment groups, inclusion or exclusion of the distal interphalangeal joints did not change the results of the trial. Scoring of the additional features did not provide additional information when considering change. In the Ratingen PsA score, the proliferation score (quantifying bony proliferation in 40 joints of hands and feet) and the disability score (quantifying destruction in the same 40 joints) proved to have a good intraobserver and interobserver variability and to be sensitive to change over a mean interval of 3 years [26]. The correlation in progression of both subscores was weak, suggesting both subscores provide additional information on progression.

Box 1. Conclusions drawn for X-ray studies in six early arthritis cohorts

Diagnosis
- Radiographs of the feet in addition to radiographs of the hands improve the sensitivity in predicting RA compared with clinical diagnosis alone.
- Periarticular decalcification is unreliable as a radiographic feature.
- Periostitis and tuft resorption do not differentiate adequately between RA and PsA. These features are not sensitive to change in PsA, at least in advanced disease. Bone proliferation in advanced PsA can be assessed reliably and is sensitive to change. It is not known whether this feature is present in early disease, and whether it can discriminate reliably between RA and PsA.
- Including distal interphalangeal joints in scores of erosions and narrowing does not improve sensitivity to change in patients with advanced PsA. It is not known whether changes in these joints differentiate between PsA and other inflammatory joint disease in patients with EIA.
- Patients with isolated abnormalities in large joints are unlikely to have RA. The contribution of abnormalities in the large joints for other diagnostic or prognostic classification is unknown.
- A substantial proportion of patients with early PsA have radiographic sacroiliitis. In patients without psoriasis and ES, it is unknown if this would contribute to classify patients within the group of SpAs.

Damage and progression of damage
- A substantial proportion of patients with EIA have erosive changes in their hands and feet and have radiographic damage that is quantifiable by classic scoring methods.
- The amount of damage and increase in damage is low, but seems to be comparable to results of more recent studies in early RA.
- In early RA, scoring methods can detect changes within 3 months if films are read in chronologic order.
- Repair in EIA has not yet been studied.
- In early RA, studying the proportion of patients whose disease becomes erosive and the increase in damage over time gives additional information.

- The relationship between disease activity, bone metabolism, and joint damage in EIA has not been resolved.

Reporting radiographic outcome in clinical trials
- The large number of zero values, low damage scores, and expected lower progression in patients who are treated early have consequences for sample sizes of patients in clinical trials.

Prognosis for functional outcome

Independent of the diagnostic value, radiographs can play a prognostic role when evaluating patients with EIA. In early RA, the predictive value of radiographic damage at baseline for future disability (defined as worse physical function [HAQ] [21], work disability [27,28], direct medical costs [29], joint surgery [30], and mortality [31]) has been well established in several longitudinal studies. In PsA, one study revealed the radiographic damage predicted mortality [32]. In EIA, Visser and colleagues [11] showed that erosions predicted persistent synovitis and progressive erosive disease. None of the EIA cohorts studied the independent prognostic value of radiographic abnormalities on functional outcome. The major bottleneck to answering this question is that long-term observations are necessary to prove this relationship reliably. In early RA, it was known that cumulative damage reflects the cumulative disease activity [33]. Increasingly, it is recognized in RA that independent pathophysiologic effects on bone metabolism have an additional role in the development of structural damage [34,35]. Nevertheless, disease activity can be used as a substitute to predict damage and functional outcome. For PsA, the role of clinical inflammation and bone metabolism to predict damage has not been addressed yet. The relationship between clinical disease activity and bone metabolism on the one hand and structural damage and functioning on the other hand might differ between diseases and needs to be studied in longer follow-up studies of patients with EIA. There are some indications to support the hypothesis that pathways other than disease activity alone contribute to structural damage in EA. In NOAR, the Larsen score at the last evaluation was only weakly explained by baseline CRP (OR of middle tertile CRP 1.5 [95% confidence interval 1–2.3] and OR of highest tertile CRP 1.1 [95% confidence interval 1.7–3.2]) [4]. In the Austrian EA Action, there was no difference in the baseline inflammatory variables between patients who developed erosive compared with nonerosive RA [6]. In the Amsterdam cohort, baseline disease activity scale (DAS) 28 was higher in patients with progressive UPA after 1 year compared with patients with mild UPA in univariate, but not in multivariate, analyses [7]. It is important to examine the relative contribution of clinical inflammation and other pathways (eg, bone metabolism) to occurrence of structural damage in EIA. This contribution would have consequences for treatment choices because there is evidence that some DCARTs have independent effects on disease activity and bone metabolism [36].

Reporting radiographic outcome in clinical trials

The large number of zero values, low damage scores, and expected lower progression in patients who are treated early have consequences for radiographic outcome in clinical trials. Landewé and van der Heijde [37] made some recommendations with regard to radiographic outcome in EIA clinical trials. Radiographic change in radiographs of hands and feet as a primary outcome is less relevant compared with the clinical outcomes. It was discussed that it could be worthwhile to stratify patients according to their likelihood to develop erosive change, but more data are needed to predict such outcomes reliably. Such strata need to be powered sufficiently to be able to measure differences.

Summary and recommendations

EIA is a clinical description preceding the classification of disease (RA, PsA, UA) or determination of the prognosis-related classification of the disease (persistent synovitis, erosive). The role of conventional radiography in the assessment of patients with EIA is to enhance such classifications. This would allow rheumatologists to apply existing knowledge about the specific conditions to the preclassification period of the disease.

Studies on conventional radiology in EIA so far have concentrated on early prediction of RA. Because most patients with EIA have self-limiting disease or progress to classic RA, the ability to predict RA is certainly relevant. However, many patients with EIA develop PsA or remain classified as having persistent UA, of which a substantial proportion are, or will become, erosive. Formal data on the prevalence of UA and outcome of these patients are lacking. It is still unknown if these patients represent a spectrum of patients with RA or a separate disease entity. Similarly, it cannot be determined whether the relationship between disease activity, radiographic damage, and functional outcome is unique for RA or universal for all inflammatory arthritides. Conclusions following the X-ray studies of six cohorts of patients who have ES (Box 1) suggest it is important to identify erosive disease in an early phase of joint inflammation.

References

[1] Gough A, Faint J, Salmon M, et al. Genetic typing of patients with inflammatory arthritis at presentation can be used to predict outcome. Arthritis Rheum 1994;37:1166–70.
[2] Masi AT. Articular patterns in the early course of rheumatoid arthritis. Am J Med 1983;75: 16–26.

[3] Kane D, Stafford L, Bresnihan B, FitzGerald O. A prospective, clinical and radiological study of early psoriatic arthritis: an early synovitis clinic experience. Rheumatology (Oxf) 2003;42: 1460–8.

[4] Bukhari M, Lunt M, Harrison BJ, et al. Rheumatoid factor is the major predictor of increasing severity of radiographic erosions in rheumatoid arthritis: results from the Norfolk Arthritis Register Study, a large inception cohort. Arthritis Rheum 2002;46:906–12.

[5] Bukhari M, Harrison B, Lunt M, et al. Time to first occurrence of erosions in inflammatory polyarthritis: results from a prospective community-based study. Arthritis Rheum 2001;44: 1248–53.

[6] Machold KP, Stamm TA, Eberl GJ, et al. Very recent onset arthritis—clinical, laboratory, and radiological findings during the first year of disease. J Rheumatol 2002;29:2278–87.

[7] Jansen LM, van Schaardenburg D, van der Horst-Bruinsma IE, Dijkmans BA. One year outcome of undifferentiated polyarthritis. Ann Rheum Dis 2002;61:700–3.

[8] Devauchelle Pensec V, Saraux A, Berthelot JM, et al. Ability of hand radiographs to predict a further diagnosis of rheumatoid arthritis in patients with early arthritis. J Rheumatol 2001; 28:2603–7.

[9] Pensec VD, Saraux A, Berthelot JM, et al. Ability of foot radiographs to predict rheumatoid arthritis in patients with early arthritis. J Rheumatol 2004;31:66–70.

[10] Plant MJ, Saklatvala J, Borg AA, et al. Measurement and prediction of radiological progression in early rheumatoid arthritis. J Rheumatol 1994;21:1808–13.

[11] Visser H, le Cessie S, Vos K, et al. How to diagnose rheumatoid arthritis early: a prediction model for persistent (erosive) arthritis. Arthritis Rheum 2002;46:357–65.

[12] Goldbach-Mansky R, Lee J, McCoy A, et al. Rheumatoid arthritis associated autoantibodies in patients with synovitis of recent onset. Arthritis Res 2000;2:236–43.

[13] Goldbach-Mansky R, Lee JM, Hoxworth JM, et al. Active synovial matrix metalloproteinase-2 is associated with radiographic erosions in patients with early synovitis. Arthritis Res 2000;2: 145–53.

[14] Rahman P, Nguyen E, Cheung C, et al. Comparison of radiological severity in psoriatic arthritis and rheumatoid arthritis. J Rheumatol 2001;28:1041–4.

[15] Harrison BJ, Silman AJ, Barrett EM, et al. Presence of psoriasis does not influence the presentation or short-term outcome of patients with early inflammatory polyarthritis. J Rheumatol 1997;24:1744–9.

[16] Punzi L, Pianon M, Rossini P, et al. Clinical and laboratory manifestations of elderly onset psoriatic arthritis: a comparison with younger onset disease. Ann Rheum Dis 1999;58:226–9.

[17] Drossaers-Bakker KW, Kroon HM, Zwinderman AH, et al. Radiographic damage of large joints in long-term rheumatoid arthritis and its relation to function. Rheumatology (Oxf) 2000; 39:998–1003.

[18] Devauchelle-Pensec V, Saraux A, Alapetite S, Colin D, Le Goff P. Diagnostic value of ra-diographs of the hands and feet in early rheumatoid arthritis. Joint Bone Spine 2002;69:434–41.

[19] van der Heijde D. Joint erosions and patients with early rheumatoid arthritis. Br J Rheumatol 1995;34(Suppl 2):74–9.

[20] Jansen LM, van Schaardenburg D, van Der Horst-Bruinsma IE, et al. Predictors of functional status in patients with early rheumatoid arthritis. Ann Rheum Dis 2000;59:223–6.

[21] Scott DL, Smith C, Kingsley G. Joint damage and disability in rheumatoid arthritis: an updated systematic review. Clin Exp Rheumatol 2003;21(Suppl 31):S20–7.

[22] Sokka T, Kautiainen H, Hakkinen A, Hannonen P. Radiographic progression is getting milder in patients with early rheumatoid arthritis: results of 3 cohorts over 5 years. J Rheumatol 2004;31: 1073–82.

[23] van der Heijde D, Dankert T, Nieman F, et al. Reliability and sensitivity to change of a simplification of the Sharp/van der Heijde radiological assessment in rheumatoid arthritis. Rheumatology (Oxf) 1999;38:941–7.

[24] Bruynesteyn K, Landewé R, Van Der Linden S, Van Der Heijde D. Radiography as primary outcome in rheumatoid arthritis: acceptable sample sizes for trials with 3 months follow-up. Ann Rheum Dis 2004;63:1413–8.

[25] Mease PJ, Kivitz AJ, Burch FX, et al. Etanercept treatment of psoriatic arthritis: safety, efficacy, and effect on disease progression. Arthritis Rheum 2004;50:2264–72.

[26] Wassenberg S, Fischer-Kahle V, Herborn G, Rau R. A method to score radiographic change in psoriatic arthritis. Z Rheumatol 2001;60:156–66.

[27] Verstappen SM, Bijlsma JW, Verkleij H, et al. Overview of work disability in rheumatoid arthritis patients as observed in cross-sectional and longitudinal surveys. Arthritis Rheum 2004; 51:488–97.

[28] Kavanaugh A, Han C, Bala M. Functional status and radiographic joint damage are associated with health economic outcomes in patients with rheumatoid arthritis. J Rheumatol 2004; 31:849–55.

[29] Verstappen SM, Verkleij H, Bijlsma JW, et al. Determinants of direct costs in Dutch rheumatoid arthritis patients. Ann Rheum Dis 2004;63:817–24.

[30] James D, Young A, Kulinskaya E, et al. Orthopaedic intervention in early rheumatoid arthritis: occurrence and predictive factors in an inception cohort of 1064 patients followed for 5 years. Rheumatology (Oxf) 2004;43:369–76.

[31] Riise T, Jacobsen BK, Gran JT. High mortality in patients with rheumatoid arthritis and atlantoaxial subluxation. J Rheumatol 2001;28:2425–9.

[32] Gladman DD, Farewell VT, Wong K, Husted J. Mortality studies in psoriatic arthritis: results from a single outpatient center: II. prognostic indicators for death. Arthritis Rheum 1998;41: 1103–10.

[33] Welsing PM, van Gestel AM, Swinkels HL, et al. The relationship between disease activity, joint destruction, and functional capacity over the course of rheumatoid arthritis. Arthritis Rheum 2001;44:2009–17.

[34] Garnero P, Geusens P, Landewé R. Biochemical markers of joint tissue turnover in early rheumatoid arthritis. Clin Exp Rheumatol 2003;21(Suppl 31):S54–8.

[35] Landewé R, Geusens P, Boers M, et al. Markers for type II collagen breakdown predict the effect of disease-modifying treatment on long-term radiographic progression in patients with rheumatoid arthritis. Arthritis Rheum 2004;50:1390–9.

[36] Lipsky PE, van der Heijde DM, St Clair EW, et al. Infliximab and methotrexate in the treatment of rheumatoid arthritis. Anti-Tumor Necrosis Factor Trial in Rheumatoid Arthritis with Concomitant Therapy Study Group. N Engl J Med 2000;343:1594–602.

[37] Landewé R, van der Heijde D. Is radiographic progression a realistic outcome measure in clinical trials with early inflammatory arthritis? Clin Exp Rheumatol 2004;21(Suppl 31):s37–41.

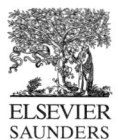

ELSEVIER
SAUNDERS

RHEUMATIC
DISEASE CLINICS
OF NORTH AMERICA

Rheum Dis Clin N Am 31 (2005) 699–714

MRI and Musculoskeletal Ultrasonography as Diagnostic Tools in Early Arthritis

Helen I. Keen, MBBS, FRACP*,
Andrew K. Brown, MBChB, MRCP(UK),
Richard J. Wakefield, BM, MRCP(UK),
Philip G. Conaghan, MBBS, PhD, FRACP, FRCP

*Academic Unit of Musculoskeletal Disease, Department of Rheumatology,
Leeds General Infirmary, Leeds, UK*

For the purpose of clinical trials, the 1987 American College of Rheumatology (ACR) [1] criteria are used to define rheumatoid arthritis (RA). These criteria have limited usefulness in clinical practice, however, with low sensitivity, particularly early in the disease process [2]. The early diagnosis of RA is crucial to long-term outcomes because it is now recognized that delaying therapy is detrimental for patient outcomes [3–5]. A major challenge is to differentiate early RA accurately from other forms of inflammatory arthritis to institute intensive therapy in a timely manner.

In clinical practice, diagnosis is largely based on the experienced clinician's interpretation of the symptoms and signs in conjunction with inflammatory markers, autoantibodies, and conventional radiography. Conventional radiography plays a significant role in the diagnosis of RA because it enables detection of the erosions characteristic of RA, which form part of the 1987 ACR criteria. The diagnostic utility of erosions in early RA is limited, however, because 70% of patients may have normal radiographs at presentation [6]. In addition, conventional radiography does not provide information about soft tissue structures or the synovium, information that may aid diagnostic and management decisions. Although conventional radiography remains an important part of early RA

---

* Corresponding author. Academic Unit of Muskuloskeletal Disease, Department of Rheumatology, Leeds General Infirmary, Great George Street, Leeds, LS1 3EX, UK.
E-mail address: hikeen@doctors.org.uk (H.I. Keen).

assessment [1], magnetic resonance imaging (MRI) and musculoskeletal ultra-sonography (MUS) are increasingly being used in rheumatology clinics for this purpose. In contrast to conventional radiography, MRI and MUS can visualize joints directly in multiple planes and gain information simultaneously about bone and soft tissue structures. This article reviews the current evidence supporting the diagnostic utility of these modalities in early RA.

Magnetic resonance imaging

MRI is an attractive imaging modality for several reasons: It provides multiplanar images and is able to visualize a range of joint structures, including synovium, tendons, ligaments, bone, and cartilage. It lacks ionizing radiation, meaning that it can be repeated at short time intervals in addition to allowing longitudinal assessment. With advances in software and sequences, development of office-based scanners, and reduction in costs, MRI is likely to become increasingly accessible.

Conventional MRI is able to assess several joints in a specific anatomic area, but may have a limited field of view (eg, only the metacarpophalangeal joints or the wrist) and is limited in clinical practice by the time it takes to perform the examination. Other relative disadvantages include the lack of portability of conventional magnets, the current limited access to machines in some countries, the need for contrast agents, and poor patient comfort factors (noise, positioning, and confined spaces). The need for prolonged immobility is a significant issue for RA patients, especially patients with early disease for whom control is not yet optimal. These properties have made MRI suitable for research and exploring proof of concept studies in RA, but may limit its usefulness in clinical practice.

Erosions

The mulitplanar nature of MRI (enabling detailed three-dimensional assess-ment of joints) and its ability to detect small cortical defects represent ideal properties for detecting bony erosions (Fig. 1). These characteristics make MRI more sensitive than conventional radiography at detecting erosions, particularly at the small joints of the hands, wrist, and feet—joints characteristically affected in early RA [7–14]. In addition, MRI is able to detect bone erosions many months before the visualization of conventional radiography erosions [12–17]. When specifically considering early RA, MRI has been shown to detect more erosive disease than conventional radiography at disease presentation and has shown that most patients have MRI erosions within months of symptom onset [15,17], even when conventional radiography is normal [17]. Two studies also have shown erosions at the metatarsophalangeal joints in early RA in the absence of radio-graphic changes in the hands and feet [13,14].

It is likely that the defects seen on MRI represent the same process as RA erosions seen on conventional radiography. Longitudinal assessment has shown

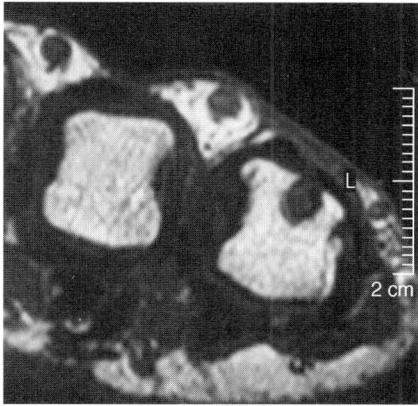

Fig. 1. MRI (T1-weighted axial section) of the right fourth and fifth metacarpophalangeal joints in a patient with rheumatoid arthritis shows a normal fourth metacarpophalangeal joint and an erosion of the fifth metacarpal head.

that erosions detected early by MRI predict the presence of conventional radiography erosions at 24 months [16]. MRI erosions are relatively specific for RA and are seen only occasionally in healthy controls [18–20]. In a 1-year study of a cohort of undifferentiated polyarthritis, MRI erosions were seen only in patients who met ACR criteria for RA at baseline or follow-up [11].

Bone edema

Bone edema refers to a unique MRI-detected abnormality with high signal intensity on fat-suppressed MRI sequences. Bone edema is defined by OMERACT as a lesion within the trabecular bone with ill-defined margins and signal characteristics of increased water content [21]. When present, it seems to be related to the severity of adjacent synovitis and seems to be a forerunner to the development of erosions [22,23]. A study imaging the wrist in early RA found bone edema to be strongly predictive of the development of conventional radiography erosions and predicting functional outcome 6 years later [23–25].

Synovitis and tenosynovitis

MRI of soft tissue structures such as synovium and tendons is enhanced by the use of the contrast agent gadolinium-diethylenetriamine pentaacetic acid (DTPA). This agent aids in the differentiation of synovial inflammation from fat and fluid (Fig. 2). Several studies have validated MRI findings of gadolinium-detected synovitis by comparing imaging findings against arthroscopy [26,27] and histopathology [26,28] and showing good correlations.

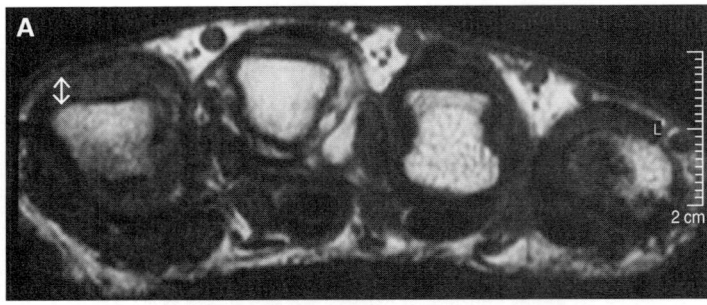

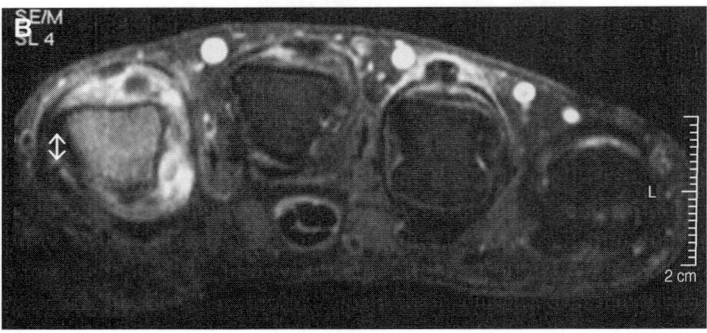

Fig. 2. MRI (T1-weighted [A] and T1 SPIR [B] postgadolinium) of the right hand metacarpopha-langeal joints in axial section of a patient with rheumatoid arthritis shows synovitis in the second metacarpophalangeal joint, flexor tenosynovitis in the third flexor tendon, and extensor tenosynovitis of the third and fourth extensor tendons.

MRI is more sensitive than clinical examination in detecting synovitis in inflammatory arthritis [7,29] and shows synovial inflammation in early RA [7,22,30,31]. Ostendorf et al [13] examined 25 patients with a clinical diagnosis of early RA that was nonerosive on conventional radiography of the hands and feet. Ten patients who had MRI of the hand revealing no OMERACT-defined pathology underwent MRI of the feet. Subclinical synovitis was detected in all 10 patients, although perhaps as expected, findings of bone edema and erosions were less common. This study provides evidence of widespread subclinical syno-vitis and bony changes in early RA that were not detected with standard assess-ments, illustrating the potential advantages of MRI in assessing disease "bulk."

The imaging of tenosynovitis, although a common pathology in RA, has been less well reported than imaging of erosions or synovitis, probably reflecting the relative importance placed on these latter pathologies. Although several studies have suggested that inflammation of tendon sheaths is commonly detected by MRI in RA [32,33], currently data on the validity of MRI-detected tenosynovitis are lacking, and there are no recommendations for MRI sequences, acquisition, or definitions. The ability of MRI to detect bony changes and synovial inflamma-tion reliably in early disease, particularly if conventional radiography is normal or clinical examination is equivocal, has implications in the diagnosis and treatment of early RA.

Diagnosis of rheumatoid arthritis

To date, data examining the utility of MRI as an aid in the diagnosis of RA are limited. Sugimoto et al [34] specifically examined the diagnostic utility of MRI in suspected early RA. Fifty patients with polyarthralgia underwent contrast-enhanced MRI of both hands and were followed for 2 years. The presence of symmetric periarticular contrast enhancement in the wrists, metacarpophalangeal joints, or proximal interphalangeal joints on MRI was found to have a sensitivity of 96% and a specificity of 86% in patients who met clinical criteria for RA. The investigators suggested an algorithm, whereby the addition of MRI criteria (symmetric periarticular enhancement) to patients with normal conventional radiography who otherwise meet the 1987 ACR criteria increases the sensitivity and specificity of the ACR criteria.

Prognostic value in early rheumatoid arthritis

MRI may have prognostic significance by providing baseline predictors of poor RA outcome. Low total MRI scores (in this study a composite of erosions, bone edema, synovitis, and tendinitis at the carpus) and absence of MRI erosions at the wrist in early RA were associated with the absence of radiographic erosive disease at 12 months [16]. MRI findings of erosions in the wrist at baseline can predict subsequent radiographic damage at 2 years [17]. It also has been shown that the proportion of MRI-detected synovitis at baseline in early RA is predictive of radiographic damage at follow-up, and that erosions are unlikely to occur in joints without synovitis [7,22,25,31,35].

In addition to predicting structural outcomes, baseline findings of bone edema and total MRI scores in early RA have been shown to correlate with functional outcomes 6 years later [24]. Identification of prognostic features at baseline by MRI in the future may allow aggressive therapy to be targeted to patients likely to have the worst outcomes.

Office-based magnetic resonance imaging

Office-based MRI machines may offer improvements in some of the problem areas of expense and patient comfort. These systems often have a low magnet strength (low field) and limited anatomic field, being able to image only a few peripheral joints using a specific sequence. The improved patient comfort may allow for more sequences to be acquired, however.

Low field MRI consistently has been found to be more sensitive to erosions than conventional radiography [36–40] in established RA. In early RA, a small study showed low field MRI to detect almost 10 times more erosions than conventional radiography [39]. Low field scanners perform similarly to conventional MRI in terms of detection of erosions and joint space narrowing [36,37]. Synovitis detection also is similar when gadolinium-DTPA is used [36]. The specificity for bone edema is high, but with only low sensitivity compared with conventional MRI [36]. Low field MRI may prove useful in the diagnosis of early RA.

Although low field MRI is less expensive than conventional MRI, there are conflicting reports as to which modality patients prefer. Verhoek et al [41] imaged the ankle and feet of more than 40 patients with a conventional scanner and a low field scanner. Unexpectedly, patient acceptance of the conventional scanner was significantly better than for the low field scanner with respect to positioning (supine position in conventional scanner compared with half-sitting position in low field scanner), examination time, and confidence in the diagnosis. There is a strong suggestion of inexperience in positioning patients, however, because the low field magnet was associated with paresthesias secondary to nerve compression in several patients. In contrast, a study comparing the two modalities imaging the hand and wrist joints found most patients preferred the low field scanner because of increased comfort, less claustrophobia, and less noise [36].

Further investigation and larger trials are required to establish the role of low field MRI in the diagnosis of early RA. The usefulness of this modality in routine clinical practice may be limited by the anatomic field, the need for contrast material to maximize the sensitivity to synovitis, and a low sensitivity to bone marrow edema (albeit of less importance). Understanding of clinical utility is required before cost can be evaluated accurately.

Monitoring outcomes

The ability of MRI to document structural progression has been documented [11,16], and when examining therapeutic interventions, MRI has been shown to be sensitive to soft tissue changes, correlating with improvements in clinical parameters of disease activity [17,42–44]. In terms of following large cohorts with long-term outcomes, the usefulness of MRI is likely to be limited by its limited anatomic field compared with conventional radiography. Bird et al [45] found that longitudinal, limited field MRI (four metacarpophalangeal joints) was not superior to conventional radiography of both hands in identifying RA progression, most likely because more joints are able to be imaged with conventional radiography.

The OMERACT MRI group was established to develop internationally recognized definitions of pathology in RA, guidelines for the interpretation of MRI data in clinical trials, and validated outcomes [21]. This initiative has provided a framework for defining objective abnormalities and damage in RA to facilitate the future use of MRI in clinical trials. A EULAR/OMERACT atlas of pathology in RA has been developed and published [46–49]. In addition, the group is addressing issues of sensitivity and reliability, particularly interreader reliability in ongoing exercises.

Musculoskeletal ultrasonography

MUS increasingly is being used in rheumatology clinics in the routine assessment of patients with inflammatory arthritis. It is relatively portable and allows dynamic, real-time assessment of multiple joints in multiple planes. Similar to MRI, MUS does not involve ionizing radiation and is suitable for repeated examination, allowing temporal information to be gathered. In contrast to MRI, MUS is a relatively quick and inexpensive procedure and can be performed in the outpatient clinic, allowing immediate correlation with the clinical presentation and providing immediate information to aid diagnosis and management. Limitations include the user-dependent nature of the modality and limited visualization of some joints. Currently, much of the research into the role of MUS in rheumatology has focused on established disease, and the role of MUS specific to early disease needs to be examined, particularly the diagnosis of early RA, so its role in the early arthritis clinic can be defined more precisely.

Erosions

Similar to MRI, the high resolution of MUS and multiplanar properties mean it is more sensitive than conventional radiography in detecting bone erosions at metacarpophalangeal, proximal interphalangeal, wrist, and metatarsophalangeal joints [9,50–53], with high levels of reproducibility (Fig. 3) [51,54]. Studies comparing erosions detected by MUS and MRI have confirmed the accuracy of MUS and shown high levels of reproducibility [9,51,55], with conflicting results as to which is more sensitive. A cross-sectional study of the metatarsophalangeal joints in established RA found that MUS detected more erosions than MRI or conventional radiography [53], whereas MRI has been shown to be more sensitive at the metacarpophalangeal joints [55]. Conversely, Magnani et al [56] examined 13 patients with early RA who had no radiographic erosions and found that MUS was as sensitive as MRI to erosions at the wrist, but detected more erosions than MRI at the metacarpophalangeal joints. MRI is generally more sensitive than MUS at erosion detection at the wrist, especially the carpus, likely owing to limited access of the MUS probe.

One of the greatest advantages of MUS over conventional radiography in the diagnosis of early RA (which generally can detect only large erosions) is the ability of MUS to detect small and large erosions. Because erosions in early RA are generally small, it is likely that MUS is likely to be of particular diagnostic use in early RA.

Synovitis and tenosynovitis

Several studies have examined the ability of MUS to detect synovitis, with validation against several other imaging techniques, including MRI, arthroscopy,

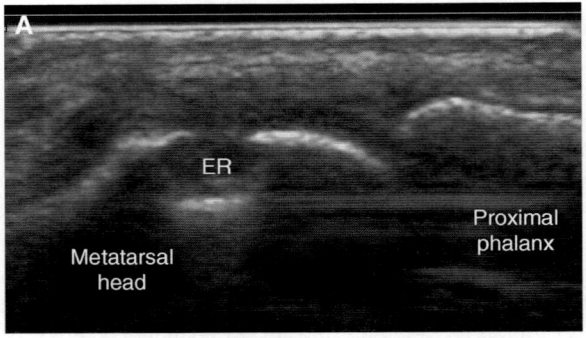

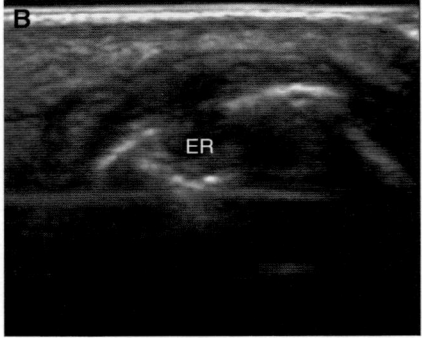

Fig. 3. US (gray-scale) shows an erosion of the lateral aspect of the fifth metatarsophalangeal joint in a patient with early rheumatoid arthritis, in longitudinal (*A*) and transverse (*B*) planes. ER, erosion.

scintigraphy, and thermography (Figs. 4 and 5) [8,57–59]. In a study examining a cohort of patients with early RA, ultrasonography was found to be more useful than MRI at identifying joint and tendon sheath effusions [55].

MUS consistently has been shown to be more sensitive than clinical examination in detecting small and large joint synovitis [53,60–62]. In a study of patients labeled as having oligoarthritis in an early arthritis clinic, MUS detected subclinical synovitis in two thirds, resulting in a revision of the diagnosis in one third [60]. This study raises important issues about disease classification, suggesting a further possible role of MUS in establishing extent of disease. Another study of 60 patients with heterogeneous knee disorders used arthroscopy as the gold standard and found MUS to be more sensitive and accurate than clinical examination [58].

The ability of MUS to detect erosions, synovitis, and tendon abnormalities accurately has potential implications in the early diagnosis and ongoing management of RA. Further work is required to determine the ability of MUS to differentiate RA from other arthritides, particularly in early disease when the clinical diagnosis is often unclear.

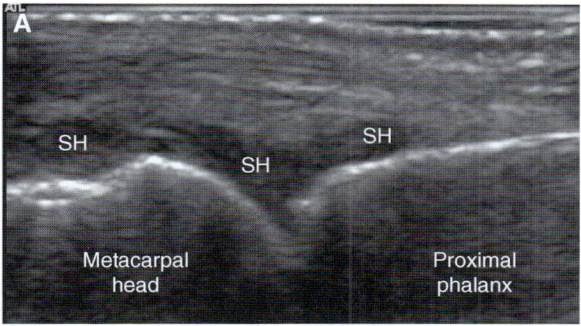

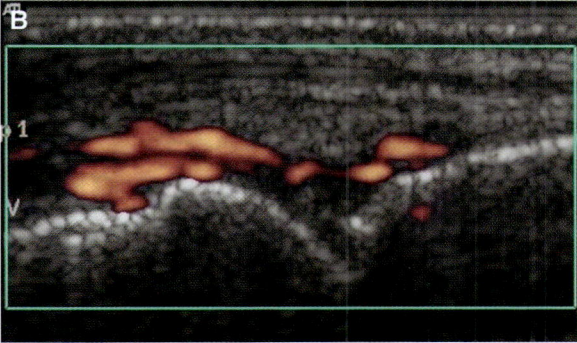

Fig. 4. US (gray-scale [A] and power Doppler [B]) shows synovial hypertrophy of the third meta-carpophalangeal joint in a patient with early rheumatoid arthritis in longitudinal plane. SH, syno-vial hypertrophy.

Power Doppler ultrasonography

The addition of power Doppler to conventional gray scale MUS allows assessment of soft tissue vascularity. Power Doppler is particularly suited to tissue with low-velocity blood flow, so it has the potential to provide additional information about vascularity of the synovium and inflammatory disease activity and to monitor temporal changes [60,63]. The technique has been validated against histopathology in the knee and seems to correlate with synovial blood vessel density [64,65]. In addition, power Doppler has been shown to correlate well with early synovial enhancement on dynamic MRI in the metacarpopha-langeal joints [66], suggesting that power Doppler is able to assess the degree of synovial inflammatory activity. Power Doppler also seems to correlate well with clinical signs of disease activity and reflect clinical improvements with treatment [67–71]. Although promising, power Doppler remains predominantly a research tool, and further investigation as to the utility and role of this modality in the management of RA is required.

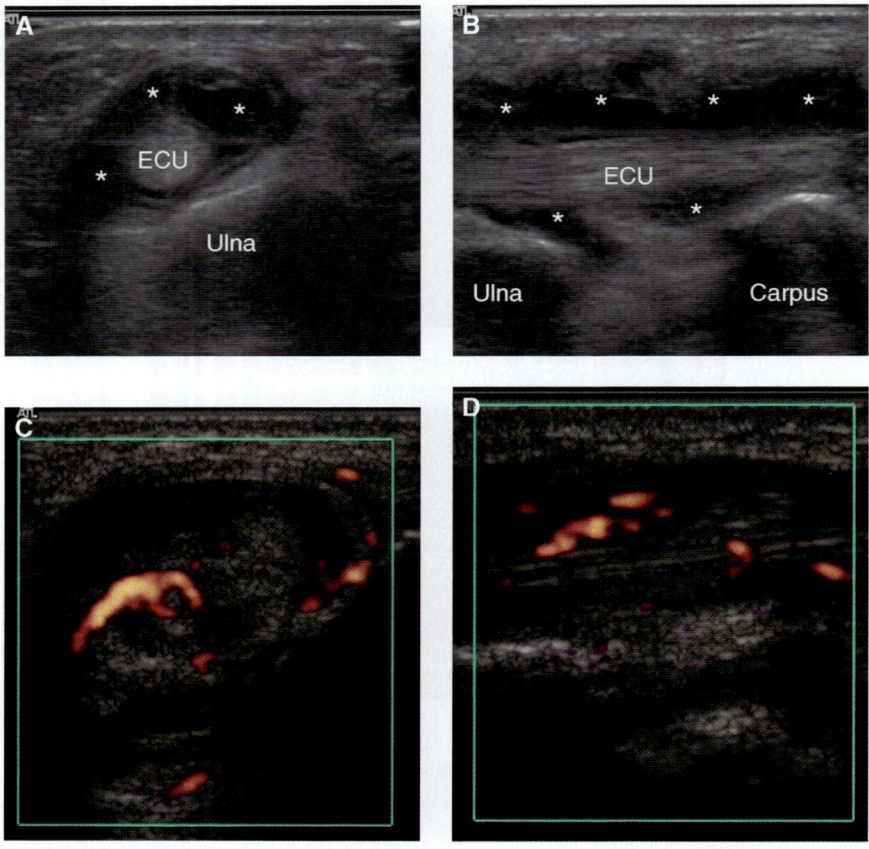

Fig. 5. US (gray-scale [A and B] and power Doppler [C and D]) shows tenosynovitis of the extensor carpi ulnaris tendon in a patient with early rheumatoid arthritis, in transverse (A and C) and longitudinal (B and D) planes. The asterisks indicate tenosynovitis. ECU, extensor carpi ulnaris tendon.

Prognositic value of musculoskeletal ultrasonography

Further investigation is required regarding the use and interpretation of MUS
findings as predictors of future outcome. A more recent study showed the
prognostic potential of MUS and power Doppler in early RA. Patients with early
erosive disease receiving stable doses of methotrexate were randomized to
receive infliximab or placebo infusions [72]. Gray scale and power Doppler were
more sensitive than traditional clinical outcome measures in discriminating between treatment groups. In the methotrexate monotherapy arm, synovial thick-
ening and vascularity shown by gray scale and power Doppler at baseline were
predictive of radiographic scores at 12 months. This study shows the potential of
MUS to predict structural outcomes and its ability to identify patients with a poor
prognosis and perhaps guide intensive therapy.

Outstanding issues

Many issues need to be addressed before MUS can be accepted as a tool for routine use in the trial and clinical setting [73,74]. As rheumatologists increasingly employ this user-dependent tool, issues of training and competency need to be addressed. There is a paucity of publications to guide training and practice of rheumatologic MUS by rheumatologists [75]. Work is currently under way, however, to develop guidelines for teaching, curricula, and competency in MUS [76–78].

With regard to reproducibility, Scheel et al [79] examined the interobserver reliability among 14 experts. Agreement was high at the shoulder, moderate at the fingers, but low at the feet. Although moderate-to-good correlation was found overall among observers, the study assessed a majority agreement only statistically—10 of the 14 experts. Other smaller studies addressed interobserver and intraobserver reliability and found good agreement, albeit between small numbers of observers [51,54,80,81]. Further validation and reproducibility studies are required. Interscanner reliability has not been addressed. There is also a paucity of publications addressing longitudinal reliability and reproducibility.

Another issue highlighted by Scheel et al [79] is the variation in methodology among observers: In their study, it was expected that observers would perform standard scans according to the guidelines of the EULAR working group for MUS. Although examinations at the knee and to a lesser extent the hands were relatively standardized, 26% of images required to examine the shoulder joint in the accepted method were not undertaken [79]. This study shows the need for standardization of MUS technique. An OMERACT ultrasound group has been established to address these issues, which need to be overcome before MUS can be accepted as a validated measurement and outcome tool [54]. The group also is working on universally agreed definitions of pathology in RA. MUS remains a promising tool in the diagnosis, monitoring, and prognosis of RA, and much work is under way to address outstanding issues.

Summary

To date, there has been much work directed at establishing the role and reliability of MUS and MRI in the management of early RA. MUS and MRI are able to augment clinical and conventional radiography findings by identifying subclinical synovitis and erosions before their detection by conventional radiography; this is true for early RA and established disease, which may allow timely and accurate diagnosis of disease, now known to be important in optimizing long-term outcomes. MRI and MUS also provide information about inflammatory activity and have the potential to identify poor prognostic features, which may allow more aggressive therapy to be targeted to patients who most need it. Further studies are required investigating the ways these modalities can be used to improve care and outcomes for patients. Both imaging modalities show promise, and similar to conventional radiography, they may become integral to the management of early RA in the future.

References

[1] Arnett F, Edworthy S, Bloch D, et al. The American Rheumatism Association 1987 revised criteria for the classification of rheumatoid arthritis. Arthritis Rheum 1988;31:315–24.

[2] Saraux A, Berthelot J, Chales G, et al. Ability of the American College of Rheumatology 1987 criteria to predict rheumatoid arthritis in patients with early arthritis and classification of these patients two years later. Arthritis Rheum 2001;44:2485–91.

[3] Mottonen T, Hannonen P, Korpela M, et al. Delay to institution of therapy and induction of remission using single-drug or combination-disease-modifying antirheumatic drug therapy in early rheumatoid arthritis. Arthritis Rheum 2002;46:894–8.

[4] Boers M, Verhoeven AC, Markusse HM, et al. Randomised comparison of combined step-down prednisolone, methotrexate and sulphasalazine with sulphasalazine alone in early rheumatoid arthritis [erratum appears in Lancet 1998 Jan 17;351:220]. Lancet 1997;350:309–18.

[5] Quinn MA, Conaghan PG, Emery P. The therapeutic approach of early intervention for rheumatoid arthritis: what is the evidence? Rheumatology 2001;40:1211–20.

[6] Emery P. Rheumatoid arthritis: not yet curable with early intensive therapy. Lancet 1997; 350:304–5.

[7] Forslind K, Ahlmen M, Eberhardt K, et al. Prediction of radiological outcome in early rheumatoid arthritis in clinical practice: role of antibodies to citrullinated peptides (anti-CCP). Ann Rheum Dis 2004;63:1090–5.

[8] Backhaus M, Kamradt T, Sandrock D, et al. Arthritis of the finger joints: a comprehensive approach comparing conventional radiography, scintigraphy, ultrasound, and contrast-enhanced magnetic resonance imaging. Arthritis Rheum 1999;42:1232–45.

[9] Backhaus M, Burmester GR, Sandrock D, et al. Prospective two year follow up study comparing novel and conventional imaging procedures in patients with arthritic finger joints. Ann Rheum Dis 2002;61:895–904.

[10] McQueen FM, Stewart N, Crabbe J, et al. Magnetic resonance imaging of the wrist in early rheumatoid arthritis reveals a high prevalence of erosions at four months after symptom onset. Ann Rheum Dis 1998;57:350–6.

[11] Klarlund M, Ostergaard M, Jensen KE, et al. Magnetic resonance imaging, radiography, and scintigraphy of the finger joints: one year follow up of patients with early arthritis. The TIRA Group. Ann Rheum Dis 2000;59:521–8.

[12] Ostergaard M, Hansen M, Stoltenberg M, et al. New radiographic bone erosions in the wrists of patients with rheumatoid arthritis are detectable with magnetic resonance imaging a median of two years earlier. Arthritis Rheum 2003;48:2128–31.

[13] Ostendorf B, Scherer A, Modder U, Schneider M. Diagnostic value of magnetic resonance imaging of the forefeet in early rheumatoid arthritis when findings on imaging of the meta-carpophalangeal joints of the hands remain normal. Arthritis Rheum 2004;50:2094–102.

[14] Boutry N, Larde A, Lapegue F, et al. Magnetic resonance imaging appearance of the hands and feet in patients with early rheumatoid arthritis. J Rheumatol 2003;30:671–9.

[15] McGonagle D, Richardson C, Green M, et al. The majority of patients with rheumatoid arthritis have erosive disease at presentation when magnetic resonance imaging of the dominant hand is employed. Arthritis Rheum 1996;39(Suppl):444.

[16] McQueen FM, Benton N, Crabbe J, et al. What is the fate of erosions in early rheumatoid arthritis? Tracking individual lesions using x rays and magnetic resonance imaging over the first two years of disease. Ann Rheum Dis 2001;60:859–68.

[17] McQueen FM, Stewart N, Crabbe J, et al. Magnetic resonance imaging of the wrist in early

rheumatoid arthritis reveals progression of erosions despite clinical improvement. Ann Rheum Dis 1999;58:156–63.

[18] Ejbjerg B, Narvestad E, Rostrup E, et al. Magnetic resonance imaging of wrist and finger joints in healthy subjects occasionally shows changes resembling erosions and synovitis as seen in rheumatoid arthritis. Arthritis Rheum 2004;50:1097–106.

[19] Tan AL, Tanner SF, Conaghan PG, et al. Role of metacarpophalangeal joint anatomic factors in the distribution of synovitis and bone erosion in early rheumatoid arthritis. Arthritis Rheum 2003;48:1214–22.

[20] McGonagle D, Conaghan PG, O'Connor P, et al. The relationship between synovitis and bone changes in early untreated rheumatoid arthritis: a controlled magnetic resonance imaging study. Arthritis Rheum 1999;42:1706–11.

[21] Ostergaard M, Peterfy C, Conaghan P, et al. OMERACT Rheumatoid Arthritis Magnetic Resonance Imaging Studies. Core set of MRI acquisitions, joint pathology definitions, and the OMERACT RA-MRI scoring system. J Rheumatol 2003;30:1385–6.

[22] Conaghan PG, O'Connor P, McGonagle D, et al. Elucidation of the relationship between synovitis and bone damage: a randomized magnetic resonance imaging study of individual joints in patients with early rheumatoid arthritis. Arthritis Rheum 2003;48:64–71.

[23] McQueen FM, Benton N, Perry D, et al. Bone edema scored on magnetic resonance imaging scans of the dominant carpus at presentation predicts radiographic joint damage of the hands and feet six years later in patients with rheumatoid arthritis. Arthritis Rheum 2003;48:1814–27.

[24] Benton N, Stewart N, Crabbe J, et al. MRI of the wrist in early rheumatoid arthritis can be used to predict functional outcome at 6 years. Ann Rheum Dis 2004;63:555–61.

[25] Savnik A, Malmskov H, Thomsen HS, et al. MRI of the wrist and finger joints in inflammatory joint diseases at 1-year interval: MRI features to predict bone erosions. Eur Radiol 2002;12:1203–10.

[26] Ostergaard M, Stoltenberg M, Lovgreen-Nielsen P, et al. Quantification of synovitis by MRI: correlation between dynamic and static gadolinium-enhanced magnetic resonance imaging and microscopic and macroscopic signs of synovial inflammation. Magn Reson Imaging 1998;16:743–54.

[27] Ostergaard M, Klarlund M, Lassere M, et al. Interreader agreement in the assessment of magnetic resonance images of rheumatoid arthritis wrist and finger joints—an international multicenter study. J Rheumatol 2001;28:1143–50.

[28] Ostergaard M, Stoltenberg M, Lovgreen-Nielsen P, et al. Magnetic resonance imaging-determined synovial membrane and joint effusion volumes in rheumatoid arthritis and osteoarthritis: comparison with the macroscopic and microscopic appearance of the synovium. Arthritis Rheum 1997;40:1856–67.

[29] Forslind K, Larsson EM, Johansson A, Svensson B. Detection of joint pathology by magnetic resonance imaging in patients with early rheumatoid arthritis. Br J Rheumatol 1997;36:683–8.

[30] Sugimoto H, Takeda A, Masuyama J, Furuse M. Early-stage rheumatoid arthritis: diagnostic accuracy of MR imaging. Radiology 1996;198:185–92.

[31] Huang J, Stewart N, Crabbe J, et al. A 1-year follow-up study of dynamic magnetic resonance imaging in early rheumatoid arthritis reveals synovitis to be increased in shared epitope-positive patients and predictive of erosions at 1 year. Rheumatology 2000;39:407–16.

[32] Hug C, Huber H, Terrier F, et al. Detection of flexor tenosynovitis by magnetic resonance imaging: its relationship to diurnal variation of symptoms. J Rheumatol 1991;18:1055–9.

[33] Valeri G, Ferrara C, Ercolani P, et al. Tendon involvement in rheumatoid arthritis of the wrist: MRI findings. Skeletal Radiol 2001;30:138–43.

[34] Sugimoto H, Takeda A, Hyodoh K. Early-stage rheumatoid arthritis: prospective study of the effectiveness of MR imaging for diagnosis. Radiology 2000;216:569–75.

[35] Savnik A, Malmskov H, Thomsen HS, et al. Magnetic resonance imaging of the wrist and finger joints in patients with inflammatory joint diseases. J Rheumatol 2001;28:2193–200.

[36] Savnik A, Malmskov H, Thomsen HS, et al. MRI of the arthritic small joints: comparison of extremity MRI (0.2 T) vs high-field MRI (1.5 T). Eur Radiol 2001;11:1030–8.

[37] Taouli B, Zaim S, Peterfy CG, et al. Rheumatoid arthritis of the hand and wrist: comparison of three imaging techniques. AJR Am J Roentgenol 2004;182:937–43.

[38] Ejbjerg B, Narvestad E, Jacobsen S, et al. Optimised, low cost, low field dedicated extremity MRI is highly specific and sensitive for synovitis and bone erosions in rheumatoid arthritis wrist and finger joints: a comparison with conventional high-field MRI and radiography. Ann Rheum Dis 2005;64(9):1280–7.

[39] Crues JV, Shellock FG, Dardashti S, et al. Identification of wrist and metacarpophalangeal joint erosions using a portable magnetic resonance imaging system compared to conventional radiographs. J Rheumatol 2004;31:676–85.

[40] Lindegaard H, Vallo J, Horslev-Petersen K, et al. Low field dedicated magnetic resonance imaging in untreated rheumatoid arthritis of recent onset. Ann Rheum Dis 2001;60:770–6.

[41] Verhoek G, Zanetti M, Duewell S, et al. MRI of the foot and ankle: diagnostic performance and patient acceptance of a dedicated low field MR scanner. J Magn Reson Imaging 1998;8:711–6.

[42] Ostergaard M, Hansen M, Stoltenberg M, et al. Magnetic resonance imaging-determined synovial membrane volume as a marker of disease activity and a predictor of progressive joint destruction in the wrists of patients with rheumatoid arthritis. Arthritis Rheum 1999;42:918–29.

[43] Reece R, Kraan M, Radjenovic A. Comparative assessment of leflunomide and methotrexate for the treatment of rheumatoid arthritis, by dynamic enhanced magnetic resonance imaging. Arthritis Rheum 1999;42:918–29.

[44] Ostergaard M, Stoltenberg M, Gideon P. Changes in synovial membrane and joint effusion volumes after intraarticular methylprednisolone: quantitative assessment of inflammatory and destructive changes in arthritis by MRI. J Rheumatol 1996;23:1151–61.

[45] Bird P, Kirkham B, Portek I, et al. Documenting damage progression in a two-year longitudinal study of rheumatoid arthritis patients with established disease (the DAMAGE study cohort): is there an advantage in the use of magnetic resonance imaging as compared with plain radiography? Arthritis Rheum 2004;50:1383–9.

[46] Conaghan P, Bird P, Ejbjerg B, et al. The EULAR-OMERACT rheumatoid arthritis MRI reference image atlas: the metacarpophalangeal joints. Ann Rheum Dis 2005;64:i11–21.

[47] Ejbjerg B, McQueen F, Lassere M, et al. The EULAR-OMERACT rheumatoid arthritis MRI reference image atlas: the wrist joint. Ann Rheum Dis 2005;64:i23–47.

[48] Ostergaard M, Edmonds J, McQueen F, et al. An introduction to the EULAR-OMERACT rheumatoid arthritis MRI reference image atlas. Ann Rheum Dis 2005;64:i3–7.

[49] Bird P, Conaghan P, Ejbjerg B, et al. The development of the EULAR–OMERACT rheumatoid arthritis MRI reference image atlas. Ann Rheum Dis 2005;64:i8–10.

[50] Weidekamm C, Koller M, Weber M, Kainberger F. Diagnostic value of high-resolution B-mode and doppler sonography for imaging of hand and finger joints in rheumatoid arthritis. Arthritis Rheum 2003;48:325–33.

[51] Wakefield RJ, Gibbon WW, Conaghan PG, et al. The value of sonography in the detection of bone erosions in patients with rheumatoid arthritis: a comparison with conventional radiography. Arthritis Rheum 2000;43:2762–70.

[52] Lopez-Ben R, Bernreuter WK, Moreland LW, Alarcon GS. Ultrasound detection of bone erosions in rheumatoid arthritis: a comparison to routine radiographs of the hands and feet. Skeletal Radiol 2004;33:80–4.

[53] Szkudlarek M, Narvestad E, Klarlund M, et al. Ultrasonography of the metatarsophalangeal joints in rheumatoid arthritis: comparison with magnetic resonance imaging, conventional radiography, and clinical examination. Arthritis Rheum 2004;50:2103–12.

[54] Szkudlarek M, Court-Payen M, Jacobsen S, et al. Interobserver agreement in ultrasonography of the finger and toe joints in rheumatoid arthritis. Arthritis Rheum 2003;48:955–62.

[55] Hoving JL, Buchbinder R, Hall S, et al. A comparison of magnetic resonance imaging, sonography, and radiography of the hand in patients with early rheumatoid arthritis. J Rheumatol 2004;31:663–75.

[56] Magnani M, Salizzoni E, Mule R, et al. Ultrasonography detection of early bone erosions in the metacarpophalangeal joints of patients with rheumatoid arthritis. Clin Exp Rheumatol 2004;22:743–8.

[57] Conaghan PG, Wakefield RJ, O'Connor P, et al. MCPJ assessment in early RA: a comparison between x-ray, MRI, high-resolution ultrasound and clinical examination. Arthritis Rheum 1998;41:S246.

[58] Karim Z, Wakefield RJ, Quinn M, et al. Validation and reproducibility of ultrasonography in the detection of synovitis in the knee: a comparison with arthroscopy and clinical examination. Arthritis Rheum 2004;50:387–94.

[59] van Holsbeeck M, van Holsbeeck K, Gevers G, et al. Staging and follow-up of rheumatoid arthritis of the knee: comparison of sonography, thermography, and clinical assessment. J Ultrasound Med 1988;7:561–6.

[60] Wakefield RJ, Green MJ, Marzo-Ortega H, et al. Should oligoarthritis be reclassified? Ultrasound reveals a high prevalence of subclinical disease. Ann Rheum Dis 2004;63:382–5.

[61] Wakefield RJ, Karim Z, Conaghan PG, et al. Sonography is more sensitive than clinical examination at detecting synovitis in the metatarsophalangeal joints than clinical examination. Arthritis Rheum 1999;42:S352.

[62] Wakefield RJ, Gibbon WW, Emery P. The current status of ultrasonography in rheumatology. Rheumatology 1999;38:195–8.

[63] Schmidt WA. Doppler sonography in rheumatology. Best Pract Res Clin Rheumatol 2004; 18:827–46.

[64] Walther M, Harms H, Krenn V, et al. Correlation of power Doppler sonography with vascularity of the synovial tissue of the knee joint in patients with osteoarthritis and rheumatoid arthritis. Arthritis Rheum 2001;44:331–8.

[65] Schmidt WA, Volker L, Zacher J, et al. Colour Doppler ultrasonography to detect pannus in knee joint synovitis. Clin Exp Rheumatol 2000;18:439–44.

[66] Szkudlarek M, Court-Payen M, Strandberg C, et al. Power Doppler ultrasonography for assessment of synovitis in the metacarpophalangeal joints of patients with rheumatoid arthritis: a comparison with dynamic magnetic resonance imaging. Arthritis Rheum 2001;44:2018–23.

[67] Terslev L, Torp-Pedersen S, Qvistgaard E, et al. Estimation of inflammation by Doppler ultrasound: quantitative changes after intra-articular treatment in rheumatoid arthritis. Ann Rheum Dis 2003;62:1049–53.

[68] Hau M, Kneitz C, Tony HP, et al. High resolution ultrasound detects a decrease in pannus vascularisation of small finger joints in patients with rheumatoid arthritis receiving treatment with soluble tumour necrosis factor alpha receptor (etanercept). Ann Rheum Dis 2002;61: 55–8.

[69] Newman JS, Laing TJ, McCarthy CJ, Adler RS. Power Doppler sonography of synovitis: assessment of therapeutic response—preliminary observations. Radiology 1996;198:582–4.

[70] Stone M, Bergin D, Whelan B, et al. Power Doppler ultrasound assessment of rheumatoid hand synovitis. J Rheumatol 2001;28:1979–82.

[71] Strunk J, Heinemann E, Neeck G, et al. A new approach to studying angiogenesis in rheumatoid arthritis by means of power Doppler ultrasonography and measurement of serum vascular endothelial growth factor. Rheumatology 2004;43:1480–3.

[72] Taylor PC, Steuer A, Gruber J, et al. Comparison of ultrasonographic assessment of synovitis and joint vascularity with radiographic evaluation in a randomized, placebo-controlled study of infliximab therapy in early rheumatoid arthritis. Arthritis Rheum 2004;50:1107–16.

[73] Ostergaard M, Wiell C. Ultrasonography in rheumatoid arthritis: a very promising method still needing more validation. Curr Opin Rheumatol 2004;16:223–30.

[74] Kane D, Balint PV, Sturrock R, Grassi W. Musculoskeletal ultrasound—a state of the art review in rheumatology: Part 1. current controversies and issues in the development of musculoskeletal ultrasound in rheumatology. Rheumatology 2004;43:823–8.

[75] Speed CA, Bearcroft PWP. Musculoskeletal sonography by rheumatologists: the challenges. Rheumatology 2002;41:241–2.

[76] Brown AK, O'Connor PJ, Wakefield RJ, et al. Practice, training, and assessment among experts performing musculoskeletal ultrasonography: toward the development of an international consensus of educational standards of ultrasonography for rheumatologists. Arthritis Rheum 2004;51:1018–22.

[77] Brown AK, O'Connor PJ, Roberts TE, et al. Recommendations for musculoskeletal ultrasonography by rheumatologists: setting global standards for best practice by expert consensus. Arthritis Rheum 2005;53:83–92.

[78] Backhaus M, Burmester GR, Gerber T, et al. Guidelines for musculoskeletal ultrasound in rheumatology. Ann Rheum Dis 2001;60:641–9.

[79] Scheel AK, Schmidt WA, Hermann KG, et al. Interobserver reliability of rheumatologists performing musculoskeletal ultrasonography: results from a EULAR "Train the Trainers" course. Ann Rheum Dis 2005;64(7):1043–9.

[80] Ribbens C, Andre B, Marcelis S, et al. Rheumatoid hand joint synovitis: gray-scale and power Doppler US quantifications following anti-tumor necrosis factor-alpha treatment: pilot study. Radiology 2003;229:562–9.

[81] Wakefield R, Ballans P, Szkudlarek M, et al. Preliminary definitions of rheumatoid arthritis pathology. J Rheumatol, in press.

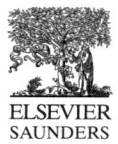

ELSEVIER
SAUNDERS

RHEUMATIC
DISEASE CLINICS
OF NORTH AMERICA

Rheum Dis Clin N Am 31 (2005) 715–728

Value of Dual-Energy X-Ray Absorptiometry as a Diagnostic and Assessment Tool in Early Rheumatoid Arthritis

Glenn Haugeberg, MD, PhD[a,b],
Paul Emery, MA, MD, FRCP[c,d],*

[a]Department of Rheumatology, Sørlandet Hospital, Kristiansand, Norway
[b]Norwegian University of Science and Technology, Trondheim, Norway
[c]Academic Unit of Musculoskeletal Disease, Rheumatology and Rehabilitation Research Unit,
Chapel Allerton Hospital, Leeds, UK
[d]Leeds Teaching Hospitals Trust, Chapel Allerton Hospital, Leeds, UK

Bone involvement in rheumatoid arthritis

Rheumatoid arthritis (RA) is a severe chronic inflammatory rheumatic disease characterized by synovitis and bone destruction. In RA, bone is affected by the involvement of erosions causing joint destruction and by osteoporosis (Fig. 1).

As early as 1865, Barwell [1] described bone involvement in RA, which later has become known as periarticular and generalized osteoporosis [2]. Periarticular osteoporosis is a typical early radiographic finding in patients who have RA and occurs mainly before erosions are visible. Periarticular osteoporosis and erosions are radiographic findings included in the revised 1987 American College of Rheumatology classification criteria for RA [3]. Generalized osteoporosis is defined as "a progressive systemic skeletal disease characterized by low bone mass and microarchitectural deterioration of bone tissue" [4]. Fractures are the only important clinical consequence.

Disease-related risk factors for generalized osteoporosis in RA include immobilization [5–8], the inflammatory process itself mediated through cytokines [5,7–9], and the use of corticosteroids (Fig. 2) [10,11].

---

* Corresponding author. Leeds Teaching Hospitals Trust, Chapel Allerton Hospital, Chapel Town Road, 2nd Floor, Leeds LS7 4SA, UK.
  E-mail address: p.emery@leeds.ac.uk (P. Emery).

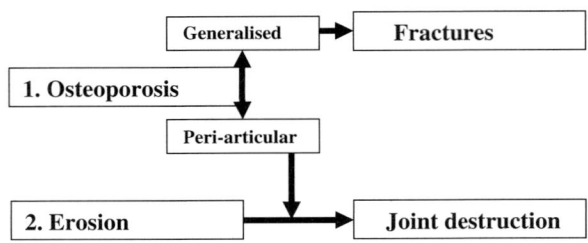

Fig. 1. Bone involvement in RA.

Protection against bone loss in RA therefore may be achieved by adequate treatment with potent antiresorptive agents (eg, bisphosphonates, hormone replacement therapy [12–14]) and by reducing the impact of disease-related risk factors for the osteoporotic process. Some studies have indicated that efficient suppression of inflammation retards or protects against accelerated generalized bone loss in RA [7,15,16].

Different underlying pathophysiologic mechanisms have been proposed for the three bone manifestations in RA. Bone erosions are considered to be caused by direct invasion by synovial pannus, periarticular osteoporosis are thought to be caused by local production of large amounts of bone-resorbing cytokines, and generalized osteoporosis is considered multifactorial with major contributions from disease activity, progressive loss of mobility, and corticosteroid use [7,17,18].

The osteoclast cell has a pivotal role in the development of erosions and of periarticular and generalized osteoporosis [19–25] in RA. Tumor necrosis factor-α and interleukin-1, which are important in the pathogenesis of synovitis in RA, have also been found to be regulators of osteoclastic bone resorbtion. This resorption is mediated through interactions with osteoprotegerin ligand (also known as receptor activator of nuclear factor κB ligand) [21,24,26]. The osteo-

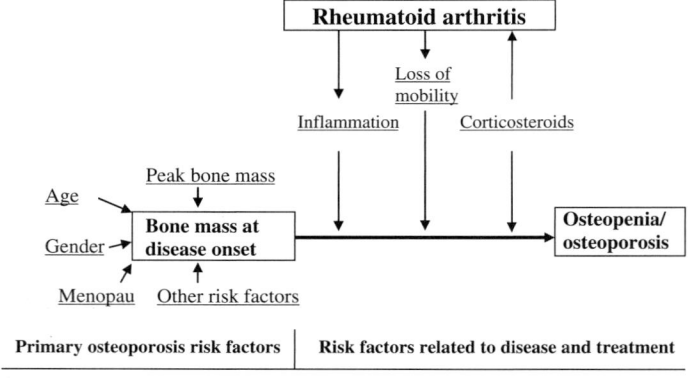

Fig. 2. Risk factors for osteoporosis in RA. (*Adapted from* Haugeberg G. Osteoporosis in rheumatoid arthritis. Tidsskr Nor Laegeforen 1997;117(5):651–4; with permission.)

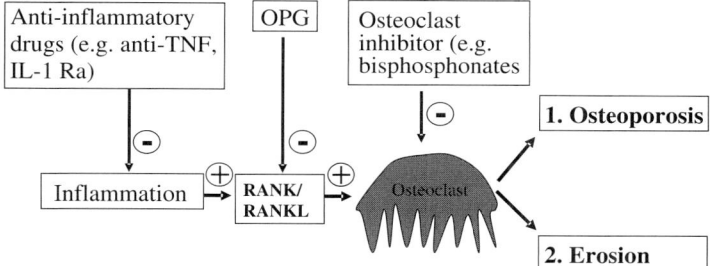

Fig. 3. Common osteoclast cellular pathway of osteoporosis and erosions in RA illustrating potential treatment strategies suppressing osteoclast activity. IL, interleukin; OPG, osteoprotegerin; TNF, tumor necrosis factor.

clast therefore seems to play the major role in the development of all three-bone manifestations in RA. This common cellular pathway suggests opportunities for both new treatment strategies (Fig. 3) and new ways of assessing patients who have inflammatory arthropathies by using measurements of bone mass.

Dual-energy x-ray absorptiometry for assessment of bone density

Bone densitometry is used primarily as a predictor of bone strength to calculate the risk of fracture [27–29] and to diagnose osteoporosis [30,31]. Because bone loss in RA is a result of the inflammatory disease process, quantitative bone measures (reflecting bone mass) may indicate the bone damaging disease process taking place, especially in early RA.

Several devices have been developed for quantitative assessment of bone mass in daily clinical practice, including dual-energy x-ray absorptiometry (DXA) [32], quantitative CT [33], radiogrammetry [34], quantitative ultrasound [35], and radiographic absorptiometry [36].

During the last 10 to 15 years, densitometry of the skeleton using DXA has become the most widespread technique for determinating bone density and is now the reference standard for assessing osteoporosis. DXA is considered precise [37–40] and accurate. In addition, DXA has a stable calibration [41] and involves only low-dose radiation [37,42,43], making DXA suitable for multiple bone mass assessments.

Because DXA measures bone density with good precision, this tool is suitable for assessment of groups and, particularly, of individuals. The in vivo short-term precision of DXA depends on the measurement site and on the DXA machine used. As shown in Table 1, the precision expressed as percentage coefficient of variation (CV%) for DXA measurement is much lower for the hand (~1%) than for the hip and spine (~2%–3%). The precision of the measurement tool is crucial in assessing individual patients, because a change must exceed the measurement error for the measurement procedure. This random measurement error, most often

Table 1
Precision and smallest detectable difference values

Location	Precision (CV%)[a]	SDD (%)[b]
Spine lombar 2–4	2.3	6.5
Hip		
Femoral neck	2.8	7.6
Total hip	1.5	4.1
Waards triangle	3.4	9.1
Trochanter	3.0	8.3
Hand	1.1	2.9

Values are based on duplicate measurements of 48 subjects measured on a Lunar Expert DXA machine (Madison, Wisconsin) (unpublished data, Department of Rheumatology, University of Leeds, Leeds, UK, 2001).

Abbreviations: CV, coefficient of variation (ratio of the SD to the mean of the measurements); SDD, smallest detectable difference.

[a] Precision expressed as a percentage of CV [45].

[b] Calculation based on the equation $2 \cdot \sqrt{2} \cdot CV(\%)$ used for SDD estimation with a level of ~95% statistical confidence [44,45].

a 95% detection limit, is called the smallest detectable difference (SDD) or least significant change. The SDD can be estimated using the formula $2 \cdot \sqrt{2} \cdot CV(\%)$ [44,45]. As shown in the Table 1, a precision of 1.1% requires a 2.9% change in bone density in the hand, whereas, for the femoral neck, a precision of 2.8% requires a change in bone mineral density (BMD) as high as 7.6% before it can be determined that a true change in bone density has taken place in an individual patient.

Measurement error can also be calculated using the method described by Bland and Altman [46]. This method is considered preferable to the use of the coefficient of variation, because this method gives an absolute and metric estimate and is independent of BMD level [45,47].

The good precision of hand BMD measurements can be improved further by using the mean values of both hands (Table 2). By using mean values of both hands, the SDD improved from a 2.6%–3.2% to a 2.1% change in hand bone density.

Table 2
Calculated precision and smallest detectable difference values for hand bone mineral density

Values	Hand bone mineral density (%)		
	Left hand	Right hand	Both hands (mean)
CV%[a]	1.14	0.92	0.75
SDD[b]	3.22	2.60	2.12

Values are based on duplicate measurements of 48 subjects measured on a Lunar Expert DXA machine (unpublished data, Department of Rheumatology, University of Leeds, Leeds, UK, 2001).

Abbreviations: CV, coefficient of variation (ratio of the SD to the mean of the measurements); SDD, smallest detectable difference.

[a] Precision expressed as a percentage of CV [45].

[b] Calculation based on the equation $2 \cdot \sqrt{2} \cdot CV(\%)$ used for SDD estimation with a level of ~95% statistical confidence [44,45].

The more precise BMD measures obtained in the hand and the higher rate of bone loss in the hand compared with the spine and hip make the hand the best site for capturing RA-related bone loss.

The next question is where to measure bone loss in the hand. Experience with hand radiographs would suggest that the periarticular regions are the best sites for detecting RA-related bone loss in the hand. These sites, however, showed high measurement errors. In a cross-sectional study of patients who had RA with average disease duration of approximately 24 months, bone loss at periarticular regions of the metacarpophalangeal joints was 23% in women and 19% in men, whereas global hand bone loss was 16% in women and 12% in men [48]. The precision of the bone measurements at these sites showed large differences, with a poor precision for the DXA bone measurements around the metacarpopha-langeal joints (ranging from 2.7% to 3.2%). For global hand measurements, the precision (expressed as coefficient of variation) was 0.9%. By applying these precision data to estimate the SDD for detection of bone loss in an individual patient, a precision error of approximately 3% requires a bone loss of approxi-mately 8% in the periarticular regions. Using the whole hand, a precision error of only 0.9% requires a bone loss of 2.5% to identify patients who have hand bone loss exceeding the measurement error of the measurement. Therefore, the greater precision of DXA measurements of the whole hand compensate for the smaller bone loss observed for whole hand as compared with DXA measurements of the periarticular regions.

Bone loss in rheumatoid arthritis: when and where?

In patients who have active RA, a significant amount of generalized skeletal bone is lost early in the disease [7], and the prevalence of osteoporosis in these patients is approximately twofold that in with the general population [6,49]. BMD loss in patients who have RA [7,50,51] has been shown to occur early in the disease process and to be more pronounced in the hands than in the hip and the lumbar spine [50,52,53]. A significant BMD reduction in patients who have RA has also been found at the distal forearm [54,55], a potential measure of periarticular osteoporosis of the wrist.

A 12-month prospective follow-up study assessing patients who had active RA with a mean disease duration of 6 months found BMD loss to be more pronounced in the hand than in hips and spine. At 12-month follow-up, BMD in the hand was reduced by 5.1%, in the femoral neck by 1.6%, in the total hip by 1.2%, and in the lumbar spine by 2.4% [56]. Mean hand BMD was measured at 3 and 6 months, in addition to the 12-month follow-up. BMD was reduced by 2.3% at 3 months and by 4.2% at 6 months.

Data suggest that the rate of bone loss in RA is highest in the first years of the disease and then slows. One study followed patients who had RA and who had been treated with nonsteroidal anti-inflammatory agents. At 1 year, the rate of hand bone loss in men was less than 5.3% in patients who had disease durations of less than 2 years and was less than 2.2% in patients who had disease durations of 2 years or longer. No hand bone loss was seen in controls [51]. For women, the corresponding data were a loss of less than 2.1% in the first 2 years and no further reduction in patients who had disease durations of 2 years or more [51]. A 5-year follow-up study (which included patients who had early RA, with durations of less than 2 years at inclusion) found the rate of DXA-measured hand bone loss to be more pronounced in the first years of the disease [57]. In this observational study of patients who had RA, loss of hand bone mass seemed to occur within the first 3 years of the 5-year period. In contrast, radiographic damage (expressed as a Larsen score) increased linearly over the 5 years [57].

Bone loss undoubtedly occurs early in the RA disease process, especially in the hand, but how early can this phenomenon be detected? This question was addressed in a study of 74 patients who had presented with onset of impaired hand function within the previous 12 months and who were suspected of having inflammatory arthritis. At baseline, all patients were classified as having undifferentiated arthritis. During follow-up 13 patients were diagnosed as having RA, 19 patients as having spondyloarthropathies or polyarthritis, and 42 patients as having a noninflammatory joint disorder. Hand bone density was reduced by less than 4.3% in the group of patients who had RA, by less than 0.5% in the spondyloarthropathy/polyarthritis group, and by less than 0.9% in the group of patients who had arthralgia [58]. No significant bone loss was seen at hip or spine in this early RA group, however.

In addition to careful clinical examination and the use of currently available laboratory and imaging data, measurement of BMD may aid in early diagnosis in patients who have previously undifferentiated arthritis.

Delay in initiating therapy with disease-modifying antirheumatic drugs can reduce treatment response in patients who have RA. Therefore, the measurement of early bone loss may be an important outcome marker [59–64].

Bone loss in rheumatoid arthritis and its association with measures of disease activity and severity

In their milestone article, Gough and colleagues [7] clearly demonstrated that generalized bone loss in RA is associated with disease activity (as measured by creatinine phosphate level) and that suppression of inflammation reduces the rate of generalized bone loss. Studies have also found that generalized bone loss is associated with other disease-related factors such as rheumatoid factor [6,65], erythrocyte sedimentation rate [66], swollen joint count [66,67], and impaired physical function [6,68,69]. Functional disability and erythrocyte sedimentation rate, but not dosage of prednisolone, were independently associated with distal radius bone density in postmenopausal patients who had RA [55].

Cross-sectional [50,52,70–72] and longitudinal studies [51] have found hand BMD loss to be strongly related to disease activity and severity early in the RA disease process.

In a 12-month follow-up study of patients presenting with undifferentiated arthritis, only mean creatinine phosphate level and positive rheumatoid factor status were found to by multivariate analysis to be independently associated with hand bone loss. This association was maintained after adjustments were made for age, health, and cumulative glucocorticoid dose using a multivariate linear regression model [58]. Suppressing inflammation by breaking the link between bone loss and inflammation therefore theoretically should stop or slow the rate of the bone loss.

Bone loss and radiographic joint damage in rheumatoid arthritis

Several studies have shown an association between radiologic joint damage and low bone mass [73–77]. Forsblad and colleagues [77] and Lodder and colleagues [74,75] found an association between hip BMD and Larsen score. Sinigaglia and colleagues [68] found that the presence of erosions is associated with a higher prevalence of osteoporosis at both the spine and hip. A 2-year follow-up study of early RA (mean disease duration of 6 months) showed that, in women, reduced BMD at onset was associated with a higher Larsen score at baseline and after 2 years [76]. The authors proposed that the development of reduced bone mass and joint destruction in RA may have a common pathophysiologic mechanism [76].

Clinical trials and cohort studies examining radiographic progression have clearly demonstrated a relationship between inflammation (disease activity) and damage [78]. It is well recognized that in early RA erosions may not be visible on conventional radiographs. During the first 1 to 2 years of follow-up, however, patients frequently develop erosions that can be seen on radiographs.

The modern imaging modalities, MR imaging and ultrasound, have been shown to be superior to radiographs in detecting erosions in early RA [79,80]. As discussed earlier, DXA measures also detect bone loss at an early stage of the disease. Preliminary data from a 48-week longitudinal study assessing patients who had RA with disease duration of less than 12 months found that, although 29% of the patients had worsened in modified Sharp score, as many as 72% had lost hand bone mass during follow-up [81]. After the measurement errors for both hand BMD-DXA measurements and for the modified Sharp score were applied, the hand-DXA method was determined to have identified more patients whose hand BMD had deteriorated than did the modified Sharp score. After 48 weeks' follow-up, only 10% of the patients had deteriorations in modified Sharp score that exceeded the SDD, whereas as many as 50% of the patients had lost hand bone mass exceeding the measurement error for DXA-measured BMD. At 24 weeks' follow-up, as many as 47% of the patients had lost hand bone mass exceeding the SDD for DXA-measured hand BMD. This finding indicates that the method is highly sensitive in identifying individual patients who have a rapid disease-related bone loss.

In comparison with radiographic joint damage scores, hand DXA provides a more sensitive tool for detecting disease-related bone damage in early RA, both in groups and in individual patients. Thus, theoretically, hand DXA may challenge the role of radiographic imaging as the reference standard for assessment of disease progression in early RA.

Bone loss as a predictor of outcome in rheumatoid arthritis

There is evidence that early changes in hand bone mass may predict both radiographic joint damage [82,83] and functional disability [57]. In a 5-year longitudinal study of patients who had early RA, early loss of hand bone mass was identified as a composite marker of disease activity and functional status and as a predictor of poor functional outcome [57]. In this study, the relative risk of poor hand functional outcome at 5 years was increased 6.9 times for patients who had hand BMD loss of 1.17 g (SDD limit) or greater compared with patients with less bone loss within the first 6 months.

There are also reports that measurements of cortical hand bone mass in the first years of RA predict subsequent radiographic joint damage [83]. Stewart and colleagues [83] found that change in cortical bone mass after 1 year was very specific (100%), with a poorer sensitivity (63%) in predicting those who either became erosive or whose erosions significantly worsened at 4 years follow-up. In another study, change in hand cortical bone mass in the first 2 years of the disease was found to be an independent predictor of progression of Sharp score at 5-year follow-up.

Bone loss measured by dual-energy x-ray absorptiometry in rheumatoid arthritis. Is this a potential new response variable to treatment effect?

Anti-inflammatory treatment with disease-modifying antirheumatic drugs and biologic agents [78] has been shown to reduce radiographic progression in RA. It has also been shown that suppression of inflammation using conventional treatment reduces the rate of generalized bone loss [7]. In a double-blind, randomized, controlled trial, BMD change in patients who had RA and who were treated with infliximab (3 mg/kg body weight) and methotrexate (n = 10) for 54 weeks was compared with methotrexate-only treatment (n = 10) [16]. In infliximab-treated patients, no bone loss was seen at the hip (<0.2%; 95% CI, −1.4, +0.9), whereas a significant bone loss was seen in the methotrexate-treated group (<2.6%; 95% CI, −4.5, −0.8). No substantial difference in hand bone loss was seen between the two groups (<2.2% versus <2.8%). The authors suggest this difference may indicate that different osteoclast-related mechanisms are involved in periarticular and generalized bone loss in RA. Another explanation may be that the infliximab doses were too low to suppress sufficiently the inflammation responsible for the RA-related hand bone loss. This hypothesis is supported by findings from a pre-study treating four patients who had active RA with infliximab, 5 mg/kg body weight. In these patients, hand bone loss was reduced by less than 1.5% (Philip P. Conaghan, MD, PhD, unpublished data, 2001).

In patients who have RA, therefore, cessation of DXA-measured hand bone loss may become the ultimate reference standard documenting complete remission and suppression of inflammation.

Bone loss in rheumatoid arthritis and its association with subsequent fractures

Compared with the general population, patients who have RA have a twofold increase in generalized osteoporosis and an increased risk of fracture. These increased risks are of clinical importance, because fractures increase morbidity [84,85] and mortality [86,87]. Specifically, patients who have RA have a two- to fourfold greater risk of hip fractures [88,89] and a two- to sixfold greater risk of vertebral fractures [90–92] than the general population. There are several identifiable risk factors in RA. In a Norwegian study of women patients aged 50–70 years who had RA, reduced BMD, long-term use of corticosteroids, and the RA itself were independently associated with vertebral deformities [90]. In another multicenter study, the Larsen radiographic joint damage score was found to be independently associated with vertebral fractures [74]. This finding is of interest, because radiographic joint damage can be considered a cumulative marker of the inflammatory disease process in RA [74]. In this study, Larsen score was independently associated with vertebral fractures even after adjusting for age, center, body mass index, and BMD. The use of corticosteroids was not independently associated with vertebral fractures, however.

Summary

In RA, bone loss, particularly in the hands, takes place early in the disease process. Hand bone loss therefore may be used for diagnosis and as a marker of early bone destruction. Bone loss is also a marker of disease activity and has the potential of being used as an outcome measure to help determine the effectiveness of treatment.

DXA is considered the reference standard. It measures bone density with high precision, making it sensitive enough to detect even small changes in bone mass and a suitable tool for assessment of individual patients. The in vivo short-term precision for DXA is dependent on the measurement site and has been shown to be better in global hand measurements than in periarticular regions or the hip or spine. Taking into account both precision and feasibility, assessment of inflammatory bone loss in early RA ideally should be performed using mean values of global hand scores. Further studies, however, are needed to validate DXA as a potential new outcome marker in early RA.

References

[1] Barwell R. Diseases of the joints. London: Harwicke; 1865.
[2] Kennedy AC, Lindsay R. Bone involvement in rheumatoid arthritis. Clin Rheum Dis 1977; 3:403–20.
[3] Arnett FC, Edworthy SM, Bloch DA, et al. The American Rheumatism Association 1987 revised criteria for the classification of rheumatoid arthritis. Arthritis Rheum 1988;31:315–24.
[4] Consensus development conference: diagnosis, prophylaxis, and treatment of osteoporosis. Am J Med 1993;94(6):646–50.
[5] Laan RF, Buijs WC, Verbeek AL, et al. Bone mineral density in patients with recent onset rheumatoid arthritis: influence of disease activity and functional capacity. Ann Rheum Dis 1993;52(1):21–6.
[6] Haugeberg G, Uhlig T, Falch JA, et al. Bone mineral density and frequency of osteoporosis in female patients with rheumatoid arthritis: results from 394 patients in the Oslo County Rheumatoid Arthritis register. Arthritis Rheum 2000;43(3):522–30.
[7] Gough AK, Lilley J, Eyre S, et al. Generalised bone loss in patients with early rheumatoid arthritis. Lancet 1994;344(8914):23–7.
[8] Eggelmeijer F, Papapoulos SE, van Paassen HC, et al. Increased bone mass with pamidronate treatment in rheumatoid arthritis. Results of a three-year randomized, double-blind trial. Arthritis Rheum 1996;39(3):396–402.
[9] Gough A, Sambrook P, Devlin J, et al. Osteoclastic activation is the principal mechanism leading to secondary osteoporosis in rheumatoid arthritis. J Rheumatol 1998;25(7):1282–9.
[10] Haugeberg G, Orstavik RE, Uhlig T, et al. Bone loss in patients with rheumatoid arthritis: results from a population-based cohort of 366 patients followed up for two years. Arthritis Rheum 2002;46(7):1720–8.
[11] Verhoeven AC, Boers M. Limited bone loss due to corticosteroids; a systematic review of prospective studies in rheumatoid arthritis and other diseases. J Rheumatol 1997;24(8): 1495–503.
[12] Boulos P, Adachi JD. Guidelines for the prevention and therapy of glucocorticoidinduced osteoporosis. Clin Exp Rheumatol 2000;18(5):S79–86.
[13] Clinical practice guidelines for the diagnosis and management of osteoporosis. Scientific Advisory Board, Osteoporosis Society of Canada. CMAJ 1996;155(8):1113–33.
[14] Recommendations for the prevention and treatment of glucocorticoid-induced osteoporosis: 2001 update. American College of Rheumatology Ad Hoc Committee on Glucocorticoid-induced Osteoporosis. Arthritis Rheum 2001;44(7):1496–503.
[15] Ferraccioli G, Casatta L, Bartoli E. Increase of bone mineral density and anabolic variables in patients with rheumatoid arthritis resistant to methotrexate after cyclosporin A therapy. J Rheumatol 1996;23(9):1539–42.
[16] Quinn M, Conaghan PG, Greenstein A, et al. The effect of TNF blockade on bone loss in early rheumatoid arthritis. Arthritis Rheum 2002;46(Suppl 9):S519.
[17] Haugeberg G. Osteoporosis in rheumatoid arthritis. Tidsskr Nor Laegeforen 1997;117(5):651–4.
[18] Sambrook P. The skeleton in rheumatoid arthritis: common mechanisms for bone erosion and osteoporosis? J Rheumatol 2000;27(11):2541–2.
[19] Sambrook PN, Eisman JA, Champion GD, et al. Determinants of axial bone loss in rheumatoid arthritis. Arthritis Rheum 1987;30(7):721–8.
[20] Goldring SR, Gravallese EM. Mechanisms of bone loss in inflammatory arthritis: diagnosis and therapeutic implications. Arthritis Res 2000;2(1):33–7.
[21] Rehman Q, Lane NE. Bone loss. Therapeutic approaches for preventing bone loss in inflammatory arthritis. Arthritis Res 2001;3(4):221–7.
[22] Gravallese EM, Manning C, Tsay A, et al. Synovial tissue in rheumatoid arthritis is a source of osteoclast differentiation factor. Arthritis Rheum 2000;43(2):250–8.
[23] Hofbauer LC, Khosla S, Dunstan CR, et al. The roles of osteoprotegerin and osteoprotegerin ligand in the paracrine regulation of bone resorption. J Bone Miner Res 2000;15(1):2–12.

[24] Takayanagi H, Iizuka H, Juji T, et al. Involvement of receptor activator of nuclear factor kappa B ligand/osteoclast differentiation factor in osteoclastogenesis from synoviocytes in rheumatoid arthritis. Arthritis Rheum 2000;43(2):259–69.

[25] Gravallese EM, Galson DL, Goldring SR, et al. The role of TNF-receptor family members and other TRAF-dependent receptors in bone resorption. Arthritis Res 2001;3(1):6–12.

[26] Redlich K, Hayer S, Maier A, et al. Tumor necrosis factor alpha-mediated joint destruction is inhibited by targeting osteoclasts with osteoprotegerin. Arthritis Rheum 2002;46(3):785–92.

[27] Gravallese EM, Goldring SR. Cellular mechanisms and the role of cytokines in bone erosions in rheumatoid arthritis. Arthritis Rheum 2000;43(10):2143–51.

[28] Cummings SR, Black DM, Nevitt MC, et al. Bone density at various sites for prediction of hip fractures. The Study of Osteoporotic Fractures Research Group. Lancet 1993;341(8837): 72–5.

[29] Marshall D, Johnell O, Wedel H. Meta-analysis of how well measures of bone mineral density predict occurrence of osteoporotic fractures. BMJ 1996;312(7041):1254–9.

[30] Black DM, Cummings SR, Genant HK, et al. Axial and appendicular bone density predict fractures in older women. J Bone Miner Res 1992;7(6):633–8.

[31] Kanis JA, Melton LJ, Christiansen C, et al. The diagnosis of osteoporosis. J Bone Miner Res 1994;9(8):1137–41.

[32] WHO Study Group. Assessment of fracture risk and its application to screening for postmenopausal osteoporosis. Geneva: World Health Organization; 1994.

[33] Blake GM, Fogelman I. Technical principles of dual energy x-ray absorptiometry. Semin Nucl Med 1997;27(3):210–28.

[34] Cann CE. Quantitative CT for determination of bone mineral density: a review. Radiology 1988;166(2):509–22.

[35] Jørgensen JT, Andersen PB, Rosholm A, et al. Digital x-ray radiogrammetry: a new appendicular bone densitometric method with high precision. Clin Physiol 2000;20(5):330–5.

[36] Njeh CF, Fuerst T, Diessel E, et al. Is quantitative ultrasound dependent on bone structure? A reflection. Osteoporos Int 2001;12(1):1–15.

[37] Bouxsein ML, Michaeli DA, Plass DB, et al. Precision and accuracy of computed digital absorptiometry for assessment of bone density of the hand. Osteoporos Int 1997;7(5):444–9.

[38] Cullum ID, Ell PJ, Ryder JP. X-ray dual-photon absorptiometry: a new method for the measurement of bone density. Br J Radiol 1989;62(739):587–92.

[39] Johnson J, Dawson-Hughes B. Precision and stability of dual-energy x-ray absorptiometry measurements. Calcif Tissue Int 1991;49(3):174–8.

[40] LeBlanc AD, Schneider VS, Engelbretson DA, et al. Precision of regional bone mineral measurements obtained from total-body scans. J Nucl Med 1990;31(1):43–5.

[41] Laan RF, van Riel PL, van de Putte LB. Bone mass in patients with rheumatoid arthritis. Ann Rheum Dis 1992;51(6):826–32.

[42] Kelly TL, Slovik DM, Neer RM. Calibration and standardization of bone mineral densitometers. J Bone Miner Res 1989;4(5):663–9.

[43] Laskey MA, Flaxman ME, Barber RW, et al. Comparative performance in vitro and in vivo of Lunar DPX and Hologic QDR-1000 dual energy x-ray absorptiometers. Br J Radiol 1991; 64(767):1023–9.

[44] Lewis MK, Blake GM, Fogelman I. Patient dose in dual x-ray absorptiometry. Osteoporos Int 1994;4(1):11–5.

[45] Genant HK, Block JE, Steiger P, et al. Appropriate use of bone densitometry. Radiology 1989;170(3 Pt 1):817–22.

[46] Ravaud P, Reny JL, Giraudeau B, et al. Individual smallest detectable difference in bone mineral density measurements. J Bone Miner Res 1999;14(8):1449–56.

[47] Bland JM, Altman DG. Statistical methods for assessing agreement between two methods of clinical measurement. Lancet 1986;1(8476):307–10.

[48] Lodder MC, Lems WF, Ader HJ, et al. Reproducibility of bone mineral density measurement in daily practice. Ann Rheum Dis 2004;63(3):285–9.

[49] Alenfeld FE, Diessel E, Brezger M, et al. Detailed analyses in periarticular osteoporosis in rheumatoid arthritis. Osteoporos Int 2000;11(5):400–7.

[50] Haugeberg G, Uhlig T, Falch JA, et al. Reduced bone mineral density in male rheumatoid arthritis patients: frequencies and associations with demographic and disease variables in ninety-four patients in the Oslo County Rheumatoid Arthritis Register. Arthritis Rheum 2000;43(12): 2776–84.

[51] Peel NF, Spittlehouse AJ, Bax DE, et al. Bone mineral density of the hand in rheumatoid arthritis. Arthritis Rheum 1994;37(7):983–91.

[52] Deodhar AA, Brabyn J, Jones PW, et al. Longitudinal study of hand bone densitometry in rheumatoid arthritis. Arthritis Rheum 1995;38(9):1204–10.

[53] Ardicoglu O, Ozgocmen S, Kamanli A, et al. Relationship between bone mineral density and radiologic scores of hands in rheumatoid arthritis. Clin Densitom 2001;4(3):263–9.

[54] Daragon A, Krzanowska K, Vittecoq O, et al. Prospective x-ray densitometry and ultra-sonography study of the hand bones of patients with rheumatoid arthritis of recent onset. Joint Bone Spine 2001;68(1):34–42.

[55] Kelly C, Bartholomew P, Lapworth A, et al. Peripheral bone density in patients with rheumatoid arthritis and factors which influence it. Eur J Intern Med 2002;13(7):423.

[56] Iwamoto J, Takeda T, Ichimura S. Forearm bone mineral density in postmenopausal women with rheumatoid arthritis. Calcif Tissue Int 2002;70(1):1–8.

[57] Conaghan P, Haugeberg G, Morton S, et al. Periarticular versus generalised bone loss in early RA. Arthritis Rheum 2002;46(Suppl):S526.

[58] Deodhar AA, Brabyn J, Pande I, et al. Hand bone densitometry in rheumatoid arthritis, a five year longitudinal study: an outcome measure and a prognostic marker. Ann Rheum Dis 2003;62(8):767–70.

[59] Haugeberg G, Green MJ, Proudman S, et al. Bone densitometry in the assessment of early inflammatory arthritis. Ann Rheum Dis 2003;62(Suppl 1):162.

[60] Bathon JM, Martin RW, Fleischmann RM, et al. A comparison of etanercept and methotrexate in patients with early rheumatoid arthritis. N Engl J Med 2000;343(22):1586–93.

[61] Bukhari MA, Wiles NJ, Lunt M, et al. Influence of disease-modifying therapy on radiographic outcome in inflammatory polyarthritis at five years: results from a large observational inception study. Arthritis Rheum 2003;48(1):46–53.

[62] Harrison B, Symmons D. Early inflammatory polyarthritis: results from the Norfolk Arthritis Register with a review of the literature. II. Outcome at three years. Rheumatology (Oxford) 2000;39(9):939–49.

[63] Landewe RB, Boers M, Verhoeven AC, et al. COBRA combination therapy in patients with early rheumatoid arthritis: long-term structural benefits of a brief intervention. Arthritis Rheum 2002;46(2):347–56.

[64] Lard LR, Visser H, Speyer I, et al. Early versus delayed treatment in patients with recent-onset rheumatoid arthritis: comparison of two cohorts who received different treatment strategies. Am J Med 2001;111(6):446–51.

[65] Machold KP, Stamm TA, Eberl GJ, et al. Very recent onset arthritis—clinical, laboratory, and radiological findings during the first year of disease. J Rheumatol 2002;29(11):2278–87.

[66] Garton MJ, Reid DM. Bone mineral density of the hip and of the anteroposterior and lateral dimensions of the spine in men with rheumatoid arthritis. Effects of low-dose corticosteroids. Arthritis Rheum 1993;36(2):222–8.

[67] Eggelmeijer F, Camps JA, Valkema R, et al. Bone mineral density in ambulant, non-steroid treated female patients with rheumatoid arthritis. Clin Exp Rheumatol 1993;11(4):381–5.

[68] van Schaardenburg D, Valkema R, Dijkmans BA, et al. Prednisone treatment of elderly-onset rheumatoid arthritis. Disease activity and bone mass in comparison with chloroquine treatment. Arthritis Rheum 1995;38(3):334–42.

[69] Sinigaglia L, Nervetti A, Mela Q, et al. A multicenter cross sectional study on bone mineral density in rheumatoid arthritis. Italian Study Group on Bone Mass in Rheumatoid Arthritis. J Rheumatol 2000;27(11):2582–9.

[70] Kroger H, Honkanen R, Saarikoski S, et al. Decreased axial bone mineral density in

perimenopausal women with rheumatoid arthritis—a population based study. Ann Rheum Dis 1994;53(1):18–23.

[71] Deodhar AA, Brabyn J, Jones PW, et al. Measurement of hand bone mineral content by dual energy x-ray absorptiometry: development of the method, and its application in normal volunteers and in patients with rheumatoid arthritis. Ann Rheum Dis 1994;53(10):685–90.

[72] Devlin J, Lilley J, Gough A, et al. Clinical associations of dual-energy x-ray absorptiometry measurement of hand bone mass in rheumatoid arthritis. Br J Rheumatol 1996;35(12):1256–62.

[73] Harrison BJ, Hutchinson CE, Adams J, et al. Assessing periarticular bone mineral density in patients with early psoriatic arthritis or rheumatoid arthritis. Ann Rheum Dis 2002;61(11): 1007–11.

[74] Sambrook P, Raj A, Hunter D, et al. Osteoporosis with low dose corticosteroids: contribution of underlying disease effects and discriminatory ability of ultrasound versus bone densitometry. J Rheumatol 2001;28(5):1063–7.

[75] Lodder MC, Haugeberg G, Lems WF, et al. Radiographic damage associated with low bone mineral density and vertebral deformities in rheumatoid arthritis: the Oslo-Truro-Amsterdam (OSTRA) collaborative study. Arthritis Rheum 2003;49(2):209–15.

[76] Lodder MC, de Jong Z, Kostense PJ, et al. Bone mineral density in patients with rheumatoid arthritis: relation between disease severity and low bone mineral density. Ann Rheum Dis 2004;63(12):1576–80.

[77] Forslind K, Keller C, Svensson B, et al. Reduced bone mineral density in early rheumatoid arthritis is associated with radiological joint damage at baseline and after 2 years in women. J Rheumatol 2003;30(12):2590–6.

[78] Forsblad DH, Larsen A, Waltbrand E, et al. Radiographic joint destruction in postmenopausal rheumatoid arthritis is strongly associated with generalised osteoporosis. Ann Rheum Dis 2003;62(7):617–23.

[79] Pincus T, Ferraccioli G, Sokka T, et al. Evidence from clinical trials and long-term observational studies that disease-modifying anti-rheumatic drugs slow radiographic progression in rheumatoid arthritis: updating a 1983 review. Rheumatology (Oxford) 2002;41(12):1346–56.

[80] Wakefield RJ, Gibbon WW, Conaghan PG, et al. The value of sonography in the detection of bone erosions in patients with rheumatoid arthritis: a comparison with conventional radiography. Arthritis Rheum 2000;43(12):2762–70.

[81] Ostergaard M, Hansen M, Stoltenberg M, et al. New radiographic bone erosions in the wrists of patients with rheumatoid arthritis are detectable with magnetic resonance imaging a median of two years earlier. Arthritis Rheum 2003;48(8):2128–31.

[82] Haugeberg G, Green MJ, Conaghan P, et al. Hand bone densitometry: the most sensitive measure detecting change in bone destruction in early rheumatoid patients. Ann Rheum Dis 2004;63(Suppl I):110.

[83] Haugeberg G, Uhlig T, Strand A, et al. Hand bone loss in rheumatoid arthritis predicts subsequent radiographic hand joint damage. Arthritis Rheum 2002;46(supplement 9):S523.

[84] Stewart A, Mackenzie LM, Black AJ, et al. Predicting erosive disease in rheumatoid arthritis. A longitudinal study of changes in bone density using digital x-ray radiogrammetry: a pilot study. Rheumatology (Oxford) 2004;43(12):1561–4.

[85] Nevitt MC, Ettinger M, Black D, et al. The association of radiographically detected vertebral fractures with back pain and function: a prospective study. Ann Intern Med 1998; 128(10):793–800.

[86] Hall SE, Criddle RA, Comito TL, et al. A case-control study of quality of life and functional impairment in women with long-standing vertebral osteoporotic fracture. Osteoporos Int 1998;9(6):508–15.

[87] Cooper C, Atkinson EJ, Jacobsen SJ, et al. Population-based study of survival after osteoporotic fractures. Am J Epidemiol 1993;137(9):1001–5.

[88] Kado DM, Browner WS, Palermo L, et al. Vertebral fractures and mortality in older women: a prospective study. Study of Osteoporotic Fractures Research Group. Arch Intern Med 1999;159(11):1215–20.

[89] Orstavik RE, Haugeberg G, Uhlig T, et al. Self reported non-vertebral fractures in rheumatoid

arthritis and population based controls: incidence and relationship with bone mineral density and clinical variables. Ann Rheum Dis 2004;63(2):177–82.

[90] Huusko TM, Korpela M, Karppi P, et al. Threefold increased risk of hip fractures with rheumatoid arthritis in Central Finland. Ann Rheum Dis 2001;60(5):521–2.

[91] Orstavik RE, Haugeberg G, Mowinckel P, et al. Vertebral deformities in rheumatoid arthritis: a comparison with population-based controls. Arch Intern Med 2004;164(4):420–5.

[92] Peel NF, Moore DJ, Barrington NA, et al. Risk of vertebral fracture and relationship to bone mineral density in steroid treated rheumatoid arthritis. Ann Rheum Dis 1995;54(10):801–6.

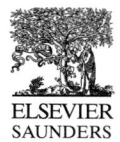

ELSEVIER
SAUNDERS

RHEUMATIC
DISEASE CLINICS
OF NORTH AMERICA

Rheum Dis Clin N Am 31 (2005) 729–744

Conventional Disease-Modifying Antirheumatic Drugs in Early Arthritis

Tuulikki Sokka, MD, PhD[a,b], Pekka Hannonen, MD, PhD[c,d],
Timo Möttönen, MD, PhD[e,f,g,*]

[a]*Department of Rheumatology, Jyväskylä Central Hospital, Jyväskylä, Finland*
[b]*Department of Rheumatology, Vanderbilt University, Nashville, TN, USA*
[c]*Kuopio University, Jyväskylä, Finland*
[d]*Department of Medicine, Jyväskylä Central Hospital, Jyväskylä, Finland*
[e]*Turku University, Turku, Finland*
[f]*Department of Medicine, Turku University Central Hospital, Turku, Finland*
[g]*Division of Rheumatology, Paimio Hospital, Paimio, Finland*

Two decades ago, rheumatoid arthritis (RA) was recognized as a disease with severe long-term consequences. Since then, a treatment strategy to relieve pain and inflammation with traditional measures [1] has changed to a strategy including aggressive treatments in early stages of the disease to prevent future damage and functional loss [2]. Gold sodium thiomalate was among the first drugs that was shown to be disease-modifying over the long-term [3], leading to one of the earliest proposals for a more active treatment strategy for early RA by Luukkainen and colleagues [4] in 1978: "...In our opinion gold treatment ought to be started in the early stages of RA, before the development of erosions. We are treating not only the actual inflammation of the joints but also the quality of the patient's life for many decades in the future." Since then, several new medications have been introduced for the treatment of RA. Currently a strategy of early, active, and continuous treatment aimed at remission is the basis of therapies for early RA.

* Corresponding author. Division of Rheumatology, Paimio Hospital, Alvar Aalto Way 275, 21540 Paimio, Finland.

E-mail address: timo.mottonen@tyks.fi (T. Möttönen).

0889-857X/05/$ – see front matter © 2005 Elsevier Inc. All rights reserved.
doi:10.1016/j.rdc.2005.07.007   *rheumatic.theclinics.com*

Conventional disease-modifying antirheumatic drugs

Several drugs with different chemical structures have been found to suppress inflammatory activity in RA and are known as "disease-modifying antirheumatic drugs" (DMARDs). These drugs differ from each other with respect to their disease-modifying properties, toxicity profiles, and survival on drug [5,6]. Some of the drugs are truly disease-modifying and have potential to slow radiographic progression in RA (Box 1) [7].

Clinical observational studies and clinical practice have shown the superiority of methotrexate versus other conventional DMARDs in the treatment of RA in terms of efficacy [7], toxicity [8,9], and drug survival [6], whereas in short-term controlled trials methotrexate seems comparable to other DMARDs [10–12]. At this time, methotrexate is the anchor drug in the treatment of early RA in many practices, primarily in the United States [13,14], which indicates a major shift in approach to RA compared with the early 1990s [6,15,16]. Many European practices used sulfasalazine, however, as the first DMARD for early RA in the 1990s [17–19].

Box 1. Conventional disease-modifying antirheumatic drugs with documented capacity to slow radiographic progression in rheumatoid arthritis

DMARDs that definitely slow radiographic progression
　　Corticosteroids
　　Cyclosporin A
　　Injectable gold salts
　　Leflunomide
　　Methotrexate
　　Sulfasalazine

DMARDs that are unlikely or may marginally slow radiographic progression
　　Azathioprine
　　Oral gold salts
　　Hydroxychloroquine
　　Penicillamine

Modified from Pincus T, Ferraccioli G, Sokka T, et al. Evidence from clinical trials and long-term observational studies that disease-modifying anti-rheumatic drugs slow radiographic progression in rheumatoid arthritis: updating a 1983 review. Rheumatology 2002;41:1346–56; with permission.

Early rheumatoid arthritis

The term "RA" is used to describe a syndrome that is capable of leading to a destructive symmetric polyarthritis and is often associated with the presence of rheumatoid factor (RF) [20]. Identification of RA in the early stages is important and difficult. Criteria for RA have been developed since 1907 [21]. Even the most recent set of criteria, the American College of Rheumatology (ACR) 1987 revised criteria [22], however, do not differentiate patients with early RA from other types of recent-onset inflammatory polyarthritides [23,24].

The time frame of early RA may range up to 5 years of symptoms in some studies [25]. Most clinical early RA cohorts define "early" as less than or equal to 6 to 24 months of disease. The median duration of symptoms at the time of enrollment was 5 to 8 months in most clinical early RA cohorts [26–28]. Very early RA has been defined with a maximum duration of symptoms of 12 weeks [29].

As noted earlier, a definite diagnosis of RA usually cannot be confirmed at early stages of the disease. It has been suggested that early inflammatory polyarthritis should not be called early RA [20]. Nevertheless, the term early RA is used in this article, recognizing that although most patients with early RA are likely to develop destructive symmetric polyarthritis, some patients may develop other diagnostic entities.

Prognosis of early rheumatoid arthritis and early therapies

Early population-based studies since the late 1950s indicated that most patients who were classified as having possible, probable, or likely RA had no evidence of disease 3 to 5 years later [30,31]. These observations may have contributed to an underestimation of RA until the severity of long-term outcomes of clinical RA was recognized in the 1980s [32,33]. In addition, in clinical early RA cohorts, most patients had severe outcomes over 15 to 40 years [34,35].

Long-term consequences of RA include joint destruction, functional decline, work disability, and early mortality [32]. Although typical for persistent disease, these characteristics are seen frequently in patients with early RA. Erosions are present in 30% of patients when first seen in the clinic [36], and most patients develop erosions during the first 2 years of disease [37–39]. Until more recently, 20% to 40% of patients with early RA became permanently work disabled over the first 2 to 3 years of the disease [40–42].

Several studies indicate that early initiation of DMARD therapy is more beneficial than late initiation [3,43–46], suggesting that a window of opportunity exists at early stages of RA [47]. Recognition of severe outcomes—and more recently evidence of benefits of early therapies—has led to the practice of starting treatment in patients with a persistent inflammatory arthritis, whether or not classification criteria of RA are met; this is provided that the patients do not meet criteria or show clinical signs of other specific arthritides (eg, crystal deposit disease, reactive arthritis, ankylosing spondylitis, psoriatic arthritis) [48]. As a result of the absence of specific prognostic markers on an individual level, some patients may be overtreated; this can be considered acceptable, however, because many of these patients may benefit from early initiation of therapies.

Early treatments for early rheumatoid arthritis in the 1970s

In 1974, a randomized controlled clinical trial [49] documented that radiographic progression over 2 years was significantly less in patients who were treated with intramuscular gold compared with patients treated with placebo. Three years later, an observational study indicated that patients treated with intramuscular gold early in the course of RA had lower radiographic progression over 5 years than patients treated with gold at later stages [3].

A Finnish cohort from Heinola was one of the first prospective cohorts with recent-onset (<6 months) RA. This cohort enrolled 103 RF-positive patients in 1973–1975 [26], who were reviewed 1, 3, 8, 15, 20, and 25 years after enrollment [50]. The treatment strategy in the Heinola cohort was early and active therapy. At the time of diagnosis, 51% of patients began gold sodium thiomalate, 31% began hydroxychloroquine, 5% began a combination of gold sodium thiomalate and hydroxychloroquine, and 2% began D-penicillamine. At the 1-year visit, 85% of patients were taking these drugs, and at the 3-year visit, 76% were still taking the drugs [51]. Most of the patients discontinued these DMARDs, however, owing to side effects or inefficacy. After 8 years, only 30% of patients were taking intramuscular gold or D-penicillamine, and 70% were taking hydroxychloroquine or no DMARDs [51,52] (Fig. 1A). Although the treatment strategy was active over the first few years, long-term benefits were reduced because of discontinuation of the drugs. Therapies could not prevent severe joint damage or amyloidosis in most patients over the subsequent 20 years [50,51,53].

"Sawtooth" strategy for early rheumatoid arthritis in the 1980s

Three different early RA cohorts were established in Finland in the 1980s. The first cohort (the 1983–1985 cohort) enrolled 58 patients (symptoms <24 months) in 1983–1985 [27], and the second cohort enrolled 77 patients (symptoms <12 months) in 1988–1989 (the 1988–1989 cohort) in Jyväskylä [28]. Another 87 patients (symptoms <24 months) were enrolled in 1986–1989 in Helsinki [54]. Although these cohorts were assembled separately with different study hypotheses, all patients were treated early, actively and continuously with traditional DMARDs, individually tailored for each patient with a goal of remission. This strategy later was termed the "sawtooth" strategy [2]. All patients also were monitored regularly to collect data for evaluation of long-term outcomes [36,42,52, 54–61].

In the 1983–1985 cohort, the first DMARD was intramuscular gold (70%) or hydroxychloroquine (30%), which was begun at the time of diagnosis (median 7 months of symptoms) [36]. The 1988–1989 cohort patients were randomized to treatments with either sulfasalazine or placebo. Because of inefficacy, placebo was replaced with intramuscular gold in 70% of patients during the first 6 months and in other placebo-treated patients by 1 year, although one patient in this cohort never received a DMARD [28,36]. The Helsinki cohort patients began intramuscular gold or sulfasalazine [54]. Other DMARDs that were given to patients in these cohorts in case of inefficacy or side effects included oral gold, azathioprine, D-penicillamine, podophyllotoxin, and later methotrexate and cyclosporine. Various combinations of these drugs also were used. Only a few patients in the 1983–1985 cohort and less than 20% of the 1988–1989 cohort took methotrexate during the first 5 years (Fig. 1B and C).

Long-term outcomes were more favorable in these cohorts compared with outcomes of previous clinical early RA cohorts. The 8-year Larsen scores of 85 RF-positive patients in the 1983–1985 and 1988–1989 cohorts who were treated according to the sawtooth strategy were significantly lower compared with the scores of 103 RF-positive patients in the Heinola cohort, most of whom discontinued intramuscular gold or hydroxychloroquine because of lack of efficacy or side effects [52]. There were undoubted differences between the two groups of patients in addition to more versus less aggressive DMARD treatment, but most probably more active treatments were beneficial concerning radiographic outcomes [7]. Functional capacity in the 1983–1985 and 1988–1989 cohorts with the median Health Assessment Questionnaire score of 0.63 at 13 years and 0.25 at 8 years in the 1997 evaluation were among the lowest published in the literature at this time [59]. Mortality was not increased in these cohorts [57,61], possibly because of more effective control of inflammation compared with previous observations in the literature [62] or because of a relatively short observation period of 8 to 14 years. Nonetheless, 20% of patients became work disabled during the first 2 years in these cohorts [42].

Although disease outcomes seem reasonably favorable in these cohorts over the first 10 years, 15- to 20-year results are needed to confirm the findings. A major lesson from RA cohort studies in the past is that of favorable 10-year outcomes versus unfavorable 20-year outcomes, as reported by Scott and colleagues [33].

Methotrexate as an anchor drug in early rheumatoid arthritis in the 1990s

The use of methotrexate for the treatment of RA increased in the 1990s [63,64]. Increased use of methotrexate, compared with the previous cohorts, was seen in the early RA cohort established in Jyväskylä in 1996–1997 [19]. In this randomized controlled study of benefits of muscle-strength exercise, patients began sulfasalazine as the first DMARD [36] and were treated according to the sawtooth strategy to aim for remission. Subsequently, after 6 months, 2 years, and

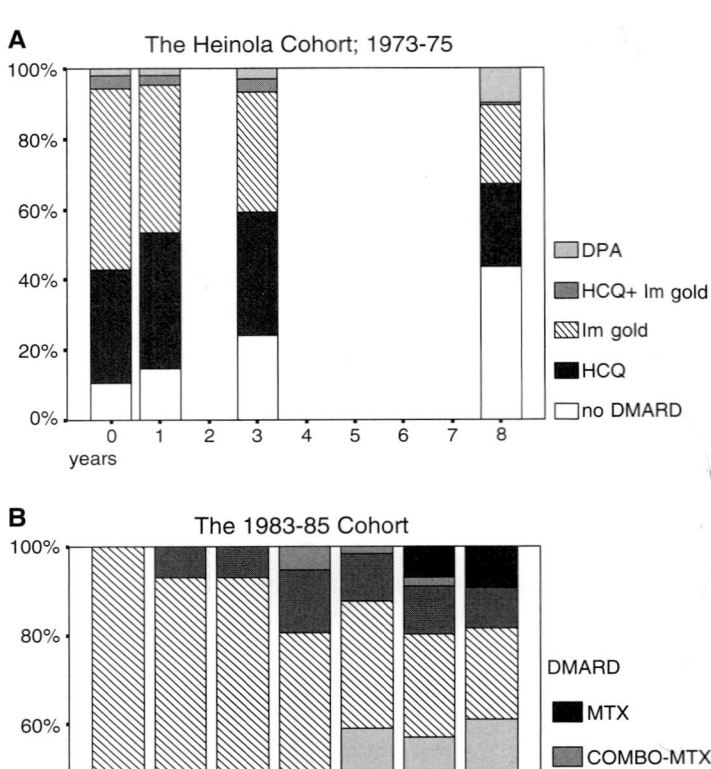

Fig. 1. (A–D) DMARDs taken by patients with early RA in four separate early RA cohorts. Percentages of patients taking each drug or combination are shown (A, *data from* Sokka T, Kaarela K, Möttönen TT, et al. Conventional monotherapy compared to a "sawtooth" treatment strategy in the radiographic progression of rheumatoid arthritis over the first eight years. Clin Exp Rheumatol 1999;17:527–32; and B–D, Sokka T, Kautiainen H, Häkkinen K, et al. Radiographic progression is getting milder in patients with early rheumatoid arthritis: results of 3 cohorts over 5 years. J Rheumatol 2004;31:1073–82.) COMBO+MTX, combination including MTX; COMBO-MTX, combination without MTX; DPA, D-penicillamine; HCQ, hydroxychloroquine, Im gold, MYO intramuscular gold; INFL, infliximab; MTX, methotrexate; SSZ, sulfasalazine.

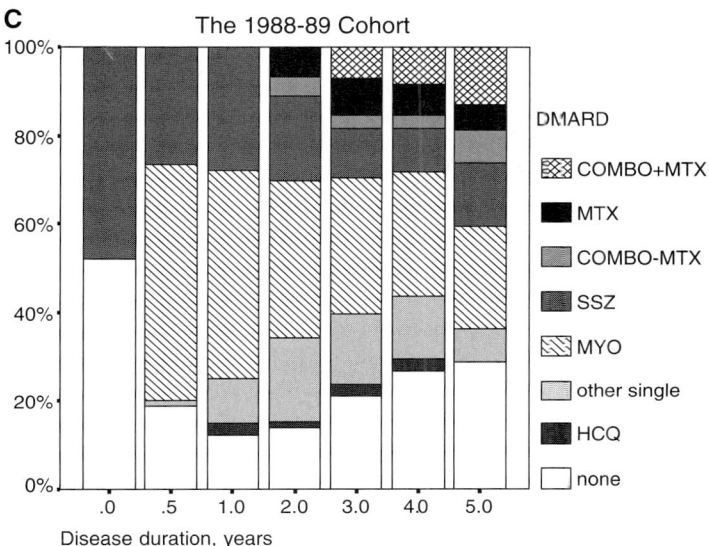

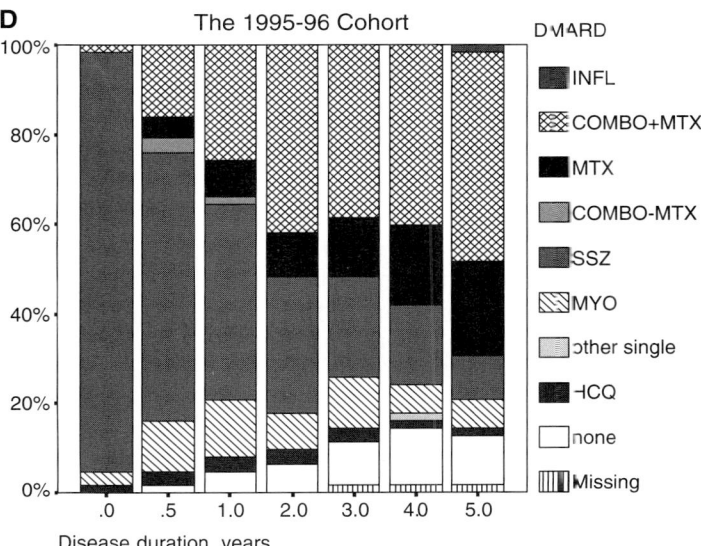

Fig. 1 (*continued*).

5 years, 24%, 50%, and 70% of patients were taking methotrexate alone or in combination with other DMARDs (Fig. 1D).

Radiographic outcomes were compared over 5 years in the 1996–1997 cohort versus the two previous Jyväskylä early RA cohorts from the 1980s. Although the proportion of patients with erosive disease was similar across the cohorts at 5 years, indicating similar potential for radiographic changes in all three cohorts, the extent of erosions according to the Larsen score was quite different. Larsen scores were lowest at 2 and 5 years in the 1996–1997 cohort [36], which most likely reflects benefits from more aggressive treatment strategies, including methotrexate as an anchor drug, although other explanations cannot be excluded [65].

Functional capacity was well maintained, with mean Health Assessment Questionnaire scores of 0.3 to 0.4 at 5 years [66]. At 2 years, 31% of patients were receiving work disability payments, however [67].

Finnish Rheumatoid Arthritis Combination Therapy Trial and evidence of superiority of early combination therapy

Eighteen Finnish rheumatology clinics participated in an investigator-initiated multicenter randomized controlled trial, the Finnish Rheumatoid Arthritis Combination Therapy Trial (FIN-RACo) [68]. This study enrolled 195 patients with early RA in 1993–1995. The patients were randomized to two treatment arms for 2 years: 97 received a combination of methotrexate, sulfasalazine, hydroxychloroquine, and prednisolone, and 98 received single-drug therapy with sulfasalazine (with or without prednisolone), in which methotrexate later was substituted in 51 patients.

The primary outcome measure of the FIN-RACo study was remission, which was defined as no tender and no swollen joints, morning stiffness lasting 15 minutes or less, no pain, and normal erythrocyte sedimentation rate. According to these strict criteria, the frequency of remission was 37% in the combination group and 18% in the single-drug group at 2 years ($P = .003$) [68]. Delay of institution of therapy played a major role in the single-drug group results. In the single-drug group, 35% of the patients with a short delay (0–4 months) were in remission at 2 years, whereas the corresponding figure in patients with a long delay (>4 months) was only 11% ($P = .021$). The frequency of remission was similar in patients with short delay (0–4 months) and long delay (>4 months) of institution of the therapy in the combination group.

The 5-year outcomes of radiographic scores and work disability favored early combination treatments, although therapies were at physicians' discretion after 2 years. The 5-year median Larsen score was 11 in the initial combination group versus 24 in the single-drug group ($P < .01$) [69]. Patients in the initial combination group were more likely to maintain their capacity to continue in paid work over 5 years compared with the single-drug group [70]. Fifty-four percent of patients who did not have ACR 20% responses over 6 months became permanently work disabled over 5 years compared with 22% of patients who had ACR 20% or 50% responses. If inflammation was controlled to a status of remission at 6 months, no patient was receiving work disability payments at 5 years [71,72]. This observation indicates that improvement rates of ACR 20% or 50% are suboptimal goals of therapies for patients with early RA.

may include remission in a few patients [93]. Because the fundamental dysregulation in RA is unknown, the term *remission* in RA encompasses continuing therapy and not a drug-free remission [94].

The remission rate of 37% at 2 years in the FIN-RACo combination group was remarkably high with a strict set of remission criteria [68] versus 18% in the single-DMARD group. In another study, only 10% of patients with early RA entered remission over 48 weeks regardless of a treatment regimen (combination of methotrexate, cyclosporine, and corticosteroids versus sulfasalazine) [95]. The combination of methotrexate, sulfasalazine, hydroxychloroquine, and prednisone seems to be remission-inducing in a third of patients with active early RA.

Further support of the observation that remission is possible in a remarkable proportion of patients with early RA comes from the Tight Control for RA (TICORA) study [96]. At 18 months, remission (according to the EULAR criteria) was met by 65% of patients who received intensive therapy, including monthly visits to a rheumatologist, assessment of disease activity to tailor therapies including DMARDs, and intra-articular and intramuscular steroids [96].

A proportion of patients with early RA do not improve with conventional treatments. In the FIN-RACo study, 20% of patients in the combination group and in the single-drug group did not meet ACR 20% at 6 months, and the percentages were 22% and 26% at 2 years [68]. In the COBRA trial, 28% of patients in the combination group and 51% in the sulfasalazine group had less than ACR 20% at 28 weeks [77]. In the TICORA study, 9% of patients in the intensive therapy group and 36% of patients in the routine therapy group had less than ACR 20% [96]. These patients with practically no response to active conventional therapies should be identified in rheumatology practices early in the disease to consider institution of biologic agents.

Summary

Treatments for early RA should aim for remission as soon as possible to avoid severe side effects of RA. Patients with early RA should be seen frequently, preferably by the same rheumatologist, to tailor therapies individually for each patient. At this time, the authors recommend a combination of methotrexate, sulfasalazine, hydroxychloroquine and prednisolone as the first treatment in patients who have active early polyarthritis; patients who have milder polyarthritis might begin methotrexate and low-dose prednisolone (5 mg/d). Biologic agents should be considered if patients do not respond to the combination treatment during the first few months.

Acknowledgments

The authors wish to thank Dr. Theodore Pincus for his helpful comments.

References

[1] Short CL, Bauer W. The course of rheumatoid arthritis in patients receiving simple medical and orthopedic measures. N Engl J Med 1948;238:142–8.

[2] Fries JF. Reevaluating the therapeutic approach to rheumatoid arthritis: the "sawtooth" strategy. J Rheumatol 1990;17(Suppl 22):12–5.

[3] Luukkainen R, Kajander A, Isomäki H. Effect of gold on progression of erosions in rheumatoid arthritis: better results with early treatment. Scand J Rheumatol 1977;6:189–92.

[4] Luukkainen R, Kajander A, Isomäki H. Treatment of rheumatoid arthritis [letter]. BMJ 1978; 2:1501.

[5] Felson DT, Anderson JJ, Meenan RF. Use of short-term efficacy/toxicity tradeoffs to select second-line drugs in rheumatoid arthritis: a meta-analysis of published clinical trials. Arthritis Rheum 1992;35:1117–25.

[6] Pincus T, Marcum SB, Callahan LF. Long-term drug therapy for rheumatoid arthritis in seven rheumatology private practices: II. Second-line drugs and prednisone. J Rheumatol 1992; 19:1885–94.

[7] Pincus T, Ferraccioli G, Sokka T, et al. Evidence from clinical trials and long-term observational studies that disease-modifying anti-rheumatic drugs slow radiographic progression in rheumatoid arthritis: updating a 1983 review. Rheumatology 2002;41:1346–56.

[8] Rau R, Schleusser B, Herborn G, Karger T. Longterm treatment of destructive rheumatoid arthritis with methotrexate. J Rheumatol 1997;24:1881–9.

[9] Yazici Y, Sokka T, Kautiainen H, et al. Long term safety of methotrexate in routine clinical care: discontinuation is unusual and rarely the result of laboratory abnormalities. Ann Rheum Dis 2005;64:207–11.

[10] Haagsma CJ, van Riel PLCM, de Jong AJL, et al. Combination of sulphasalazine and methotrexate versus the single components in early rheumatoid arthritis: a randomized, controlled, double-blind, 52 week clinical trial. Br J Rheumatol 1997;36:1082–8.

[11] Dougados M, Combe B, Cantagrel A, et al. Combination therapy in early rheumatoid arthritis: a randomized, controlled, double blind 52 week clinical trial of sulphasalazine and methotrexate compared to single components. Ann Rheum Dis 1999;58:220–5.

[12] Felson DT, Anderson JJ, Meenan RF. The comparative efficacy and toxicity of second-line drugs in rheumatoid arthritis: results of two metaanalyses. Arthritis Rheum 1990;33:1449–61.

[13] Sokka T, Pincus T. Contemporary disease modifying antirheumatic drugs (DMARD) in patients with recent onset rheumatoid arthritis in a US private practice: methotrexate as the anchor drug in 90% and new DMARD in 30% of patients. J Rheumatol 2002;29:2521–4.

[14] Paulus HE, Bulpitt KJ, Ramos B, et al. Relative contributions of the components of the American College of Rheumatology 20% criteria for improvement to responder status in patients with early seropositive rheumatoid arthritis. Arthritis Rheum 2000;43:2743–50.

[15] Ward MM, Fries JF. Trends in antirheumatic medication use among patients with rheumatoid arthritis, 1981–1996. J Rheumatol 1998;25:408–16.

[16] Mikuls TR. The changing face of rheumatoid arthritis therapy: results of serial surveys. Arthritis Rheum 2000;43:464–7.

[17] Wiles NJ, Lunt M, Barrett EM, et al. Reduced disability at five years with early treatment of inflammatory polyarthritis: results from a large observational cohort, using propensity models to adjust for disease severity. Arthritis Rheum 2001;44:1033–42.

[18] Papadopoulos NG, Alamanos Y, Papadopoulos IA, et al. Disease modifying antirheumatic drugs in early rheumatoid arthritis: a longterm observational study. J Rheumatol 2002;29:261–6.

[19] Häkkinen A, Sokka T, Kotaniemi A, et al. A randomized two-year study of the effects of dynamic strength training on muscle strength, disease activity, functional capacity, and bone mineral density in early rheumatoid arthritis. Arthritis Rheum 2001;44:515–22.

[20] Symmons DPM, Hazes JMW, Silman AJ. Cases of early inflammatory polyarthritis should not be classified as having rheumatoid arthritis. J Rheumatol 2003;30:902–4.

[21] Allbutt TC, Rolleston HD. A system of medicine. London: Macmillan; 1907.

[22] Arnett FC, Edworthy SM, Bloch DA, et al. The American Rheumatism Association 1987 revised criteria for the classification of rheumatoid arthritis. Arthritis Rheum 1988;31:315–24.

[23] Harrison BJ, Symmons DPM, Barrett EM, et al. The performance of the 1987 ARA classification criteria for rheumatoid arthritis in a population based cohort of patients with early inflammatory polyarthritis. J Rheumatol 1998;25:2324–30.

[24] Saraux A, Berthelot JM, Chalès G, et al. Ability of the American College of Rheumatology 1987 criteria to predict rheumatoid arthritis in patients with early arthritis and classification of these patients two years later. Arthritis Rheum 2001;44:2485–91.

[25] Helliwell PS, O'Hara M, Holdsworth J, et al. A 12-month randomized controlled trial of patient education on radiographic changes and quality of life in early rheumatoid arthritis. Rheumatology (Oxf) 1999;38:303–8.

[26] Kaarela K. Prognostic factors and diagnostic criteria in early rheumatoid arthritis. Scand J Rheumatol 1985;57(Suppl):1–54.

[27] Möttönen TT. Prediction of erosiveness and rate of development of new erosions in early rheumatoid arthritis. Ann Rheum Dis 1988;47:648–53.

[28] Hannonen P, Möttönen T, Hakola M, et al. Sulfasalazine in early rheumatoid arthritis. Arthritis Rheum 1993;36:1501–9.

[29] Machold KP, Stamm TA, Eberl GJ, et al. Very recent onset arthritis—clinical, laboratory, and radiological findings during the first year of disease. J Rheumatol 2002;29:2278–87.

[30] Mikkelsen WM, Dodge H. A four year follow-up of suspected rheumatoid arthritis: the Tecumseh, Michigan, community health study. Arthritis Rheum 1969;12:87–91.

[31] O'Sullivan JB, Cathcart ES. The prevalence of rheumatoid arthritis: follow-up evaluation of the effect of criteria on rates in Sudbury, Massachusetts. Ann Intern Med 1972;76:573–7.

[32] Pincus T, Callahan LF, Sale WG, et al. Severe functional declines, work disability, and increased mortality in seventy-five rheumatoid arthritis patients studied over nine years. Arthritis Rheum 1984;27:864–72.

[33] Scott DL, Symmons DP, Coulton BL, et al. Long-term outcome of treating rheumatoid arthritis: results after 20 years. Lancet 1987;16:1108–11.

[34] Palm TM, Kaarela K, Hakala MS, et al. Need and sequence of large joint replacements in rheumatoid arthritis: a 25-year follow-up study. Clin Exp Rheumatol 2002;20:392–4.

[35] Minaur N, Jacoby R, Cosh J, et al. Outcome after 40 years with rheumatoid arthritis: a prospective study of function, disease activity and mortality. J Rheumatol 2004;31:3–8.

[36] Sokka T, Kautiainen H, Häkkinen K, et al. Radiographic progression is getting milder in patients with early rheumatoid arthritis: results of 3 cohorts over 5 years. J Rheumatol 2004;31:1073–82.

[37] Brook A, Corbett M. Radiographic changes in early rheumatoid disease. Ann Rheum Dis 1977; 36:71–3.

[38] Fuchs HA, Kaye JJ, Callahan LF, et al. Evidence of significant radiographic damage in rheumatoid arthritis within the first 2 years of disease. J Rheumatol 1989;16:585–91.

[39] Lindqvist E, Jonsson K, Saxne T, et al. Course of radiographic damage over 10 years in a cohort with early rheumatic arthritis. Ann Rheum Dis 2003;62:611–6.

[40] Eberhardt KB, Fex E. Functional impairment and disability in early rheumatoid arthritis—development over 5 years. J Rheumatol 1995;22:1037–42.

[41] Mau W, Bornmann M, Weber H, et al. Prediction of permanent work disability in a follow-up study of early rheumatoid arthritis: results of a tree structured analysis using RECPAM. Br J Rheumatol 1996;35:652–9.

[42] Sokka T, Kautiainen H, Möttönen T, et al. Work disability in rheumatoid arthritis 10 years after the diagnosis. J Rheumatol 1999;26:1681–5.

[43] Egsmose C, Lund B, Borg G, et al. Patients with rheumatoid arthritis benefit from early 2nd line therapy: 5 year followup of a prospective double blind placebo controlled study. J Rheumatol 1995;22:2208–13.

[44] Munro R, Hampson R, McEntegart A, et al. Improved functional outcome in patients with early rheumatoid arthritis treated with intramuscular gold: results of a five year prospective study. Ann Rheum Dis 1998;57:88–93.

[45] Möttönen T, Hannonen P, Korpela M, et al. Delay to institution of therapy and induction of remission using single-drug or combination-disease-modifying antirheumatic drug therapy in early rheumatoid arthritis. Arthritis Rheum 2002;46:894–8.

[46] Nell VP, Machold KP, Eberl G, et al. Benefit of very early referral and very early therapy with disease-modifying anti-rheumatic drugs in patients with early rheumatoid arthritis. Rheumatology (Oxf) 2004;43:906–14.

[47] Emery P. Therapeutic approaches for early rheumatoid arthritis. How early? How aggressive? Br J Rheumatol 1995;34(Suppl 2):87–90.

[48] Makinen H, Kautiainen H, Hannonen P, et al. Frequency of remissions in early rheumatoid arthritis defined by three sets of criteria: a 5-year follow-up study. J Rheumatol 2005;32(5): 796–800.

[49] Sigler JW, Bluhm GB, Duncan H, et al. Gold salts in the treatment of rheumatoid arthritis: a double-blind study. Ann Intern Med 1974;80:21–6.

[50] Sokka T. Early rheumatoid arthritis in Finland. Clin Exp Rheumatol 2003;21:S133–7.

[51] Jantti JK, Kaarela K, Belt EA, Kautiainen HJ. Incidence of severe outcome in rheumatoid arthritis during 20 years. J Rheumatol 2002;29:688–92.

[52] Sokka TM, Kaarela K, Möttönen TT, et al. Conventional monotherapy compared to a "sawtooth" treatment strategy in the radiographic procession of rheumatoid arthritis over the first eight years. Clin Exp Rheumatol 1999;17:527–32.

[53] Kaarela K, Kautiainen H. Continuous progression of radiological destruction in seropositive rheumatoid arthritis. J Rheumatol 1997;24:1285–7.

[54] Peltomaa R, Leirisalo-Repo M, Helve T, et al. Effect of age on 3 year outcome in early rheumatoid arthritis. J Rheumatol 2000;27:638–43.

[55] Möttönen T, Paimela L, Ahonen J, et al. Outcome in patients with early rheumatoid arthritis treated according to the "sawtooth" strategy. Arthritis Rheum 1996;39:996–1005.

[56] Möttönen T, Paimela L, Leirisalo-Repo M, et al. Only high disease activity and positive rheumatoid factor indicate poor prognosis in patients with early rheumatoid arthritis treated with "sawtooth" strategy. Ann Rheum Dis 1998;57:533–9.

[57] Sokka T, Möttönen T, Hannonen P. Mortality in early "sawtooth" treated rheumatoid arthritis patients during the first 8–14 years. Scand J Rheumatol 1999;28:282–7.

[58] Sokka T, Hannonen P. Utility of disease modifying antirheumatic drugs in "sawtooth" strategy: a prospective study of early rheumatoid arthritis patients up to 15 years. Ann Rheum Dis 1999;58:618–22.

[59] Sokka T, Möttönen T, Hannonen P. Disease-modifying anti-rheumatic drug use according to the 'sawtooth' treatment strategy improves the functional outcome in rheumatoid arthritis: results of a long-term follow-up study with review of the literature. Rheumatology 2000;39:34–42.

[60] Peltomaa R, Paimela L, Helve T, et al. Effect of treatment on the outcome of very early rheumatoid arthritis. Scan J Rheumatol 2001;30:143–8.

[61] Peltomaa R, Paimela L, Kautiainen H, et al. Mortality in patients with rheumatoid arthritis treated actively from the time of diagnosis. Ann Rheum Dis 2002;61:889–94.

[62] Pincus T, Callahan LF, Vaughn WK. Questionnaire, walking time and button test measures of functional capacity as predictive markers for mortality in rheumatoid arthritis. J Rheumatol 1987;14:240–51.

[63] Sokka TM, Kautiainen HJ, Hannonen PJ. A retrospective study of treating RA patients with various combinations of slow-acting antirheumatic drugs in a county hospital. Scand J Rheumatol 1997;26:440–3.

[64] Klaukka T, Kaarela K. Methotrexate is the leading DMARD in Finland. Ann Rheum Dis 2003; 62:494–6.

[65] Walji S, Bykerk VP. Rheumatoid arthritis: is the disease becoming milder or is treatment improving? J Rheumatol 2004;31:1023–5.

[66] Hakkinen A, Sokka T, Hannonen P. A home-based two-year strength training period in early rheumatoid arthritis led to good long-term compliance: a five-year followup. Arthritis Rheum 2004;51:56–62.

[67] Hakkinen A, Sokka T, Lietsalmi AM, et al. Effects of dynamic strength training on physical function, Valpar 9 work sample test, and working capacity in patients with recent-onset rheumatoid arthritis 3. Arthritis Rheum 2003;49:71–7.

[68] Möttönen T, Hannonen P, Leirisalo-Repo M, et al. Comparison of combination therapy with single-drug therapy in early rheumatoid arthritis: a randomised trial. FIN-RACo trial group. Lancet 1999;353:1568–73.

[69] Korpela M, Laasonen L, Hannonen P, et al. Retardation of joint damage in patients with early rheumatoid arthritis by initial aggressive treatment with disease-modifying antirheumatic drugs: five-year experience from the FIN-RACo study. Arthritis Rheum 2004;50:2072–81.

[70] Puolakka K, Kautiainen H, Mottonen T, et al. Impact of initial aggressive drug treatment with a combination of disease-modifying antirheumatic drugs on the development of work disability in early rheumatoid arthritis: a five-year randomized followup trial. Arthritis Rheum 2004;50: 55–62.

[71] Puolakka K, Kautiainen H, Möttönen T, et al. Predictors of productivity loss in early rheumatoid arthritis: a 5 year follow up study. Ann Rheum Dis 2005;64:130–3.

[72] Puolakka K, Kautiainen H, Möttönen T, et al. Early suppression of disease activity is essential for maintenance of work capacity in patients with recent-onset rheumatoid arthritis: five-year experience from the FIN-RACo trial. Arthritis Rheum 2005;52:36–41.

[73] Pincus T, Sokka T, Stein CM. Are long-term very low doses of prednisone for patients with rheumatoid arthritis as helpful as high doses are harmful? Ann Intern Med 2002;136:76–8.

[74] Pincus T, Sokka T, Kautiainen H. Patients seen for standard rheumatoid arthritis care have significantly better articular, radiographic, laboratory, and functional status in 2000 than in 1985. Arthritis Rheum 2005;52(4):1009–19.

[75] Möttönen T, Hannonen P, Leirisalo-Repo M, et al for FIN-RACo-trial group. Combination therapy in rheumatoid arthritis. Lancet 1999;354:952.

[76] van Everdingen AA, Jacobs JWG, van Reesema DRS, et al. Low-dose prednisone therapy for patients with early active rheumatoid arthritis: clinical efficacy, disease-modifying properties, and side effects. Ann Intern Med 2002;136:1–12.

[77] Boers M, Verhoeven AC, Markusse HM, et al. Randomised comparison of combined step-down prednisolone, methotrexate and sulphasalazine with sulphasalazine alone in early rheumatoid arthritis. Lancet 1997;350:309–18.

[78] Emery P, Salmon M. Early rheumatoid arthritis: time to aim for remission? Ann Rheum Dis 1995;54:944–7.

[79] Weinblatt ME. Rheumatoid arthritis: treat now, not later! [editorial]. Ann Intern Med 1996; 124:773–4.

[80] Pincus T, Stein CM, Wolfe F. "No evidence of disease" in rheumatoid arthritis using methotrexate in combination with other drugs: a contemporary goal for rheumatology care? Clin Exp Rheumatol 1997;15:591–6.

[81] Yelin E, Meenan R, Nevitt M, et al. Work disability in rheumatoid arthritis: effects of disease, social, and work factors. Ann Intern Med 1980;93:551–6.

[82] Mäkisara GL, Mäkisara P. Prognosis of functional capacity and work capacity in rheumatoid arthritis. Clin Rheumatol 1982;1:117–25.

[83] Fex E, Larsson B, Nived K, et al. Effect of rheumatoid arthritis on work status and social and leisure time activities in patients followed 8 years from onset. J Rheumatol 1998;25:44–50.

[84] Krause D, Schleusser B, Herborn G, et al. Response to methotrexate treatment is associated with reduced mortality in patients with severe rheumatoid arthritis. Arthritis Rheum 2000;43:14–21.

[85] Choi HK, Hernán MA, Seeger JD, et al. Methotrexate and mortality in patients with rheumatoid arthritis: a prospective study. Lancet 2002;359:1173–7.

[86] Wolfe F, Ross K, Hawley DJ, et al. The prognosis of rheumatoid arthritis and undifferentiated polyarthritis syndrome in the clinic: a study of 1141 patients. J Rheumatol 1993;20:2005–9.

[87] Prevoo ML, van Gestel AM, van't Hof MA, et al. Remission in a prospective study of patients with rheumatoid arthritis: American Rheumatism Association preliminary remission criteria in relation to the disease activity score. Br J Rheumatol 1996;35:1101–5.

[88] Balsa A, Carmona L, Gonzalez-Alvaro I, et al. Value of Disease Activity Score 28 (DAS28) and DAS28-3 compared to American College of Rheumatology-defined remission in rheumatoid arthritis. J Rheumatol 2004;31:40–6.

[89] Sokka T, Pincus T. Most patients receiving routine care for rheumatoid arthritis in 2001 did not meet inclusion criteria for most recent clinical trials or American College of Rheumatology criteria for remission. J Rheumatol 2003;30:1138–46.

[90] Suarez-Almazor ME, Soskolne CL, Saunders LD, et al. Outcome in rheumatoid arthritis: a 1985 inception cohort study. J Rheumatol 1994;21:1438–46.

[91] Young A, Dixey J, Cox N, et al. How does functional disability in early rheumatoid arthritis (RA) affect patients and their live? Results of 5 years of follow-up in 732 patients from the Early RA Study (ERAS). Rheumatol 2000;39:603–11.

[92] Lindqvist E, Saxne T, Geborek P, et al. Ten year outcome in a cohort of patients with early rheumatoid arthritis: health status, disease process, and damage. Ann Rheum Dis 2002;61:1055–9.

[93] Pincus T, Callahan LF. How many types of patients meet classification criteria for RA? J Rheumatol 1994;21:1385–9.

[94] ten Wolde S, Breedveld FC, Hermans J, et al. Randomised placebo-controlled study of stopping second-line drugs in rheumatoid arthritis. Lancet 1996;347:347–52.

[95] Proudman SM, Conaghan PG, Richardson C, et al. Treatment of poor-prognosis early rheumatoid arthritis: a randomized study of treatment with methotrexate, cyclosporin A, and intraarticular corticosteroids compared with sulfasalazine alone. Arthritis Rheum 2000;43:1809–19.

[96] Grigor C, Capell H, Stirling A, et al. Effect of a treatment strategy of tight control for rheumatoid arthritis (the TICORA study): a single-blind randomised controlled trial. Lancet 2004;364:263–9.

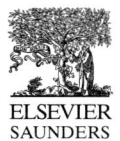
RHEUMATIC
DISEASE CLINICS
OF NORTH AMERICA

ELSEVIER
SAUNDERS

Rheum Dis Clin N Am 31 (2005) 745–762

Biologics in Early Rheumatoid Arthritis

Jeska K. de Vries-Bouwstra, MD[a,*],
Ben A.C. Dijkmans, MD, PhD[a],
Ferdinand C. Breedveld, MD, PhD[b,c]

[a]*Department of Rheumatology, VU University Medical Center, Amsterdam, The Netherlands*
[b]*Department of Rheumatology, Leiden University Medical Center, Leiden, The Netherlands*
[c]*Department of Internal Medicine, Leiden University Medical Center, Leiden, The Netherlands*

Rheumatoid arthritis (RA) is a systemic autoimmune disease characterized by chronic inflammation of the synovial joints resulting in joint damage and loss of function. The consequences of RA can vary from hardly any impairment to severe disease with continuing high disease activity and progressive joint destruction resulting in severe functional decline and increased mortality [1–3]. The ultimate goal in managing RA is to prevent joint damage and to maintain functional ability. Evidence shows that substantial and irreversible joint damage already occurs within the first 2 years after disease onset [4]. Current clinical practice is to treat earlier and more aggressively and is resulting in remarkably improved outcome of RA patients [5–8]. Treatment with a combination of disease-modifying antirheumatic drugs (DMARDs), with or without prednisone, early in the disease course has been shown to be highly effective in slowing progression of joint damage [9–12]. Intensive monitoring of disease activity and adjusting DMARD use accordingly have resulted in 65% of RA patients achieving remission [13]. These findings are important because it has been shown that patients with persistent disease activity continue to develop joint damage and to lose functional capacity, which is directly related to increased morbidity and mortality [1–3].

Among the new therapeutic approaches to RA, the introduction of biologic agents has established complete new standards for treatment of RA. The term *biologics* refers to a group of therapeutic agents that modify the biologic re-

---

* Corresponding author. Department of Rheumatology C1R, Leiden University Medical Center, PO Box 9600, 2300 RC, Leiden, The Netherlands.
E-mail address: jkdevriesbouwstra@lumc.nl (J.K. de Vries-Bouwstra).

rheumatic.theclinics.com

sponses as observed in the pathophysiologic inflammatory process in RA [14]. Although traditional DMARDs generally slow joint damage progression, the prevention of joint damage has become a revolutionary possibility, particularly with the biologics inhibiting tumor necrosis factor (TNF)-α. Currently, infliximab, etanercept, and adalimumab, all inhibiting TNF-α, are registered for treatment of RA. These TNF-α inhibitors suppress disease activity directly and powerfully and lower the disease burden significantly from the moment that treatment is started [15–17]. Anakinra, a recombinant form of the naturally occurring interleukin-1 receptor antagonist, also is registered to treat RA. The clinical and radiologic effectiveness of anakinra is less convincing, however, compared with the effectiveness of the TNF-α inhibitors, and, to date, no trials with anakinra for early, DMARD-naïve RA have been published [18]. In contrast, numerous trials studying the effectiveness of infliximab, etanercept, and adalimumab in early RA have been performed.

It has been shown that a brief intervention early in the course of RA can "reset" radiologic progression rates during subsequent years independent of consequent therapy [11]. In addition, delayed treatment trials have shown that a delay of only 3 to 9 months in starting DMARD therapy has a significant negative impact on radiographic outcome 2 years later [6,9]. Both these observations support the existence of a "window of opportunity": a period in early-stage RA during which the progression rate of joint damage is set, and therapeutic interventions can exert maximum effects. Because the TNF-α inhibitors have been proved to stop joint damage progression in severe progressive RA, the achievements of these agents in early RA are currently of great interest. This article describes and discusses current knowledge for the use of TNF-α inhibitors in early RA.

Infliximab

Infliximab (cA2 MAb, Remicade) is a chimeric human/mouse monoclonal antibody against TNF-α consisting of human IgG1 and murine Fv that binds with high affinity and specificity to human, soluble and membrane bound TNF-α [14,18]. Infliximab is administered intravenously, and the distribution is mainly intravascular with half-life of 8 to 12 days. Treatment of RA with infliximab has been developed and approved in combination with methotrexate.

The effectiveness of infliximab has been proved by results of clinical trials evaluating the additional effect of infliximab to methotrexate compared with placebo in active long-standing RA [19,20]. The Anti-TNF Trial in Rheumatoid Arthritis with Concomitant Therapy (ATTRACT) [16,20,21] showed that the combination of infliximab and methotrexate was superior to methotrexate alone for clinical and radiologic outcome at weeks 30 and 54. This study included 428 patients with active RA despite treatment with methotrexate in a minimum dose of 12.5 mg/wk, who were allocated randomly to receive placebo or one of four regimens of infliximab: 3 mg/kg or 10 mg/kg, every 4 or every 8 weeks. For the subgroup of 82 patients with early RA (disease duration ≤3 years), these results were comparable. A further subset analysis of these 82 patients with early RA was performed to evaluate radiographic damage at week 102 [22]. Compared with all ATTRACT patients, these early RA patients had lower baseline Sharp van der Heijde scores (SHS) (median total score 18 compared with 51.5), but higher predicted annual progression rate (median 11.3 compared with 7.3). Radiographs were available for 61 of 82 patients: 12 patients receiving methotrexate and placebo and 49 patients receiving methotrexate and infliximab. Early RA patients receiving methotrexate alone showed significant progression of radiologic damage (median total ΔSHS 14.3), whereas progression of joint damage was almost totally inhibited in early RA patients receiving the combination of methotrexate and infliximab (median total ΔSHS 0.5). The progression rate in the early RA group receiving methotrexate alone was higher compared with the progression rate in all patients in the ATTRACT study receiving methotrexate alone. In the early RA patients receiving methotrexate and infliximab, the progression of radiologic damage was comparable to all patients receiving the combination, with the lowest infliximab dose regimen being equally effective as the higher doses of infliximab. Given the small sample size and the nature of the analysis, conclusions based on this study must be limited. Nevertheless, the results of this subanalysis indicate that the additional effect of infliximab is even greater in patients with early RA compared with patients with long-standing disease.

Placebo-controlled studies of infliximab in early rheumatoid arthritis

In November 2004, the results of a double-blind, placebo-controlled trial comparing the combination infliximab and methotrexate with methotrexate alone in early RA (≤3 years) were published [23]. A total of 1049 methotrexate-naive patients with active disease (≥10 swollen joints, ≥12 tender joints, and at least one of the following: rheumatoid factor positivity, radiographic erosions of the hands or feet, or C-reactive protein [CRP] ≥2 mg/dL) were included. At baseline, mean disease duration was 0.9 year, and more than 80% of patients had erosive disease. All patients received methotrexate, 20 mg/wk, combined with either placebo or infliximab, 3 mg/kg, or infliximab, 6 mg/kg, infusions at 0, 2, and 6 weeks and thereafter every 8 weeks until week 46. After 54 weeks of follow-up, patients treated with the combination methotrexate and 3 mg/kg or 6 mg/kg of infliximab showed a higher percentage of overall American College of Rheumatology (ACR) improvement from baseline compared with patients receiving placebo (median 38.9% and 46.7% compared with 26.4%; $P < .001$). Among patients receiving infliximab the percentages fulfilling ACR 20, ACR 50, ACR 70, and ACR 90 were significantly higher compared with placebo. For placebo, ACR 20 was 53.6%, ACR 50 was 32.1%, ACR 70 was 21.2%, and ACR 90 was 6.6%. For infliximab, 3 mg/kg, ACR 20 was 62.4%, ACR 50 was 45.6%, ACR 70 was 32.5%, and ACR 90 was 10%; for infliximab, 6 mg/kg, ACR 20 was 66.2%, ACR 50 was 50.4%, ACR 70 was 37.2%, and ACR 90 was 16.9% (Table 1). The percentage of patients achieving remission (DAS 28<2.6) was

Table 1
Efficacy of methotrexate, tumor necrosis factor–inhibitors and the combination tumor necrosis factor–inhibitor and methotrexate in early rheumatoid arthritis

| Trial | | | Population | | | Clinical outcome (% of patients) | | | | Radiologic outcome |
Name [Ref.]	Type	Comparison	Follow-up (wk)	No. of patients	Disease duration	Regimen	ACR50	ACR70	Remission (DAS₂₈ < 2.6)	ΔSHS[a] (mean)
Aspire [23]	RCT	MTX alone vs. MTX + infliximab	54	1049	≥ 3 mo and ≤ 3 y	MTX + placebo	32	21	15	3.7
						MTX + IFX 3 mg/kg	46*	33**	21***	0.4*
						MTX + IFX 6 mg/kg	50*	37*	31*	0.5*
TEMPO [30]	Subanalysis of RCT	MTX + etanercept vs. either drug alone	104	229 (of 682)	≥ 6 mo and ≤ 3 y	MTX + placebo	43	23	19	—
						Etanercept + placebo	58	33	34	—
						MTX + etanercept	69****	44****	43	—
PREMIER [39]	RCT	MTX + adalimumab vs. either drug alone	104	799	< 3 y	MTX	43	28	25	10.4
						Adalimumab	37	27	25	5.5******
						MTX + adalimumab	59*****	47*****	50*****	1.9*****

Abbreviations: MTX, methotrexate; RCT, randomized controlled trial.

[a] Progression of joint damage as measured with Sharp-Van der Heijde score.

* P < 0.001 compared to MTX + placebo; ** P = 0.002 compared to MTX + placebo; *** P = 0.065 compared to MTX + placebo; **** P < 0.05 compared to MTX alone; ***** P < 0.001 compared to MTX alone and to adalimumab alone; ****** P < 0.001 compared to MTX alone.

significantly higher in the patients receiving infliximab: 15% for placebo compared with 21% for infliximab, 3 mg/kg, and 31% for infliximab, 6 mg/kg. Mean total progression of radiologic joint damage (SHS) was 3.7 for the placebo group, 0.4 for the infliximab, 3mg/kg, group and 0.5 for the infliximab, 6 mg/kg, group ($P<.001$). In the placebo group, 11% of patients ($n=31$) showed progression greater than the smallest detectable difference ($\Delta SHS > 9.03$); in the infliximab, 3 mg/kg, group, 3.9% ($n=14$), and in the infliximab, 6 mg/kg, group, 1.9% ($n=7$) ($P<.001$ for placebo compared with either infliximab group). Compared with patients receiving methotrexate alone, the combination with infliximab resulted in an additional 11% of patients improving at least 0.22 points in the Health Assessment Questionnaire (HAQ) score, which is set as a clinically relevant improvement. The proportion of patients with one or more serious adverse events was higher in the methotrexate and infliximab group (14%) than in the methotrexate and placebo group (11%) with significantly more serious infections (2.1% versus 5.6% and 5% for placebo; infliximab, 3 mg/kg, and infliximab, 6 mg/kg). In particular, community-acquired pneumonia occurred more frequently in the patients receiving infliximab, with an observed incidence of 2% compared with 0% for placebo.

The results of this study show the additional clinical, functional, and radiologic benefits of methotrexate and infliximab compared with methotrexate alone in patients with early RA with a poor prognosis. Beneficial effects of methotrexate monotherapy also were underlined with 65% of these patients showing a clinically relevant improvement of functional ability (HAQ score) and with a median progression of erosions of 0.3 point. Given the study population with highly active RA, the higher percentage of serious infections in the infliximab group, and the observed benefits of methotrexate monotherapy, this study does not absolutely prove the superiority of the combination with infliximab for all individual patients with early RA.

To investigate the possibility of monitoring of treatment success in terms of joint damage, Taylor and colleagues [24] performed a placebo-controlled randomized clinical trial in 24 patients with early RA with ultrasound assessments at week 18 to predict the development of joint damage after 1 year of treatment with infliximab. Eligible patients had symptoms for a maximum of 3 years, were IgM rheumatoid factor positive, had at least one erosion in a metacarpophalangeal joint, and were treated with oral methotrexate for at least 8 weeks, in a stable dose (12.5–17.5 mg/wk). All patients received infusions at weeks 0, 2, and 6 and then every 8 weeks until week 46, 12 patients with infliximab, 5 mg/kg, and 12 patients with placebo. Methotrexate was continued at baseline dose until week 18. Thereafter, methotrexate was increased to a maximum of 25 mg/wk if a 50% reduction in number of swollen joints in the hands and wrists was not achieved. The mean disease duration of included patients was 1.5 years, with a mean duration of treatment with methotrexate (mean dose 15 mg/wk) of 11 months. At week 18, there was a significant higher reduction of synovial thickness in the infliximab group (-50% versus $+1.2\%$; $P=.014$). After 54 weeks, progression of total SHS was greater in the patients receiving placebo compared with the patients receiving infliximab (median 14 [interquartile range 17] versus median 3.3 [interquartile range 3.3]; $P = .056$). At week 54, patients in the infliximab group showed a moderate or good clinical response (DAS 28 and ACR response levels) more often, without the need to increase methotrexate dosage (median total increase of methotrexate 0 mg/wk compared with 6.3 mg/wk in the placebo group; $P = .001$). Remarkably, correlations of baseline synovial thickness and baseline synovial vascularity with progression of SHS were strongly positive in the placebo group, but weakly negative and nonsignificant in the infliximab group. These results suggest that patients with early RA and high baseline disease activity may benefit most from treatment with infliximab with respect to progression of radiologic damage, and that indicators for poor prognosis at baseline are overruled by treatment with infliximab.

Infliximab as remission-induction therapy

Some small studies have been performed to test the hypothesis whether early treatment with TNF-α inhibitors in early RA patients with poor prognosis results in sustained improvement of outcome. Conaghan and colleagues [25] conducted a pilot study in five patients with newly diagnosed RA to investigate whether high-dose induction therapy with infliximab results in long-term, drug-free remission. Included patients had a mean symptom duration of 7.3 months, were DMARD-naïve, and fulfilled three or more criteria for poor prognosis. Patients were treated with methotrexate, 15 mg/ wk, combined with infliximab, 10 mg/kg at weeks 0, 2, 6, and 10 with an optional extra infusion at week 12 if remission was not achieved. After the initial four infusions, remission was achieved in one patient, three patients showed highly significant improvement (two ACR 70% response and one ACR 50% response), and one patient showed no improvement. One additional infusion did not result in further clinical improvement, and drug-free remission was achieved in none of the patients.

A double-blind, placebo-controlled study was performed in 20 DMARD-naïve patients with early RA with poor prognosis (mean symptom duration of 6 months) [26]. All patients were treated with methotrexate combined with either placebo or infliximab, 3mg/kg, during 1 year, and patients were followed in an open-label fashion for another year. Patients receiving infliximab showed significantly greater reduction of synovitis as measured by MRI of the second through fifth metacarpophalangeal joints ($t = 4$, 14 and 54 weeks), a lower erosion score ($t = 54$ weeks), and better functional improvement (HAQ; $t = 54$ weeks). After a mean of 90 weeks of follow-up (ie, after a mean of 44 weeks without infliximab), none of the patients fulfilling ACR 50 response at $t = 54$ weeks (78%) had experienced a flare of disease activity (median DAS $28 < 2.6$). This study indicates that by starting treatment with a combination of methotrexate and infliximab, sustained clinical improvement can be achieved even after stopping infliximab. That these results are not fully confirmed by the study of Conaghan and colleagues [25] can be explained partly by the differences in treatment period and outcome measures (drug-free remission versus ACR 50 response).

Etanercept

Etanercept (TNFR:Fc, Enbrel) is a dimeric recombinant fusion protein consisting of the extracellular portion of the human p75-TNF receptor type II and the Fc portion of a type 1 human immunoglobulin (IgG1). Etanercept acts as a competitive inhibitor of TNF by binding primarily soluble TNF-α and TNF-β. Etanercept has a half-life of ±3 days and is administered subcutaneously twice weekly. It is registered as monotherapy for RA [14,18].

The clinical efficacy and safety of etanercept were shown in several randomized, double-blind, and placebo-controlled trials in patients with active RA despite DMARD treatment [27,28]. These trials generally showed that etanercept is well tolerated and results in rapid and sustained clinical and functional improvement, also when added to methotrexate. A head-to-head comparison of the combination etanercept and methotrexate with either drug alone was performed, the Trial of Etanercept and Methotrexate with Radiographic Patient Outcomes (TEMPO) [17]. This double-blind, placebo-controlled trial comprising 682 patients with active RA and disease duration between 6 months and 20 years (mean 6.6 years) showed that the combination was superior to either drug alone. Included patients had previously failed on at least one DMARD other than methotrexate and received etanercept, 25 mg twice weekly; oral methotrexate, 7.5 mg/wk to 20 mg/wk; or the combination. After 1 year, the percentage of patients achieving ACR 50 and ACR 70 responses was consistently and significantly higher in the combination group compared with each other group. At week 52, 35% of the patients receiving the combination achieved clinical remission (DAS <1.6) compared with 13% of the patients on methotrexate and 16% of the patients on etanercept. The progression of joint damage over 52 weeks was lowest in the combination group, with a significant lowering of total SHS compared with baseline. Evaluation of the progression of radiologic damage over 2 years in 622 patients with at least one follow-up x-ray showed lack of progression of total SHS (Δ SHS $\leq$0.5) in 60%, 68%, and 78% of patients in the methotrexate, etanercept, and combination groups. The combination therapy resulted in sustained and significant lowering of total SHS compared with baseline, suggesting that repair of damage is possible with the combination methotrexate and etanercept [29].

Of all patients participating in the TEMPO trial, approximately 30% had at baseline a disease duration of less than 3 years. After 2 years of follow-up, a post hoc analysis was performed to evaluate the therapeutic effect of the combination of etanercept and methotrexate ($n = 77$) compared with either drug alone ($n = 77$ for etanercept and $n = 75$ for methotrexate) in patients with early-stage RA [30]. Patients receiving the combination showed significantly higher clinical response and better functional improvement compared with patients receiving either methotrexate or etanercept. The proportion of patients achieving ACR 50 was 43%, 58%, and 69%, and the proportion of patients achieving ACR 70 was 23%, 33%, and 44% for methotrexate, etanercept, and the combination (see Table 1). Remission (DAS <1.6) was achieved in 19% of the patients on methotrexate, in

34% of the patients on etanercept and in 43% of the patients on the combination. Overall, therapeutic responses of early RA patients were comparable to the responses of all patients participating in the TEMPO trial.

Altogether these results strongly suggest that the combination of methotrexate and etanercept is superior to etanercept monotherapy, especially with respect to the measurements indicating excellent clinical responses (ACR 50, ACR 70, DAS remission and complete absence of radiologic progression). The subanalysis in early RA patients did not show additional benefits of the combination for this group of patients.

Randomized controlled trial with etanercept in early rheumatoid arthritis

The Early Rheumatoid Arthritis (ERA) trial is the first clinical trial designed and performed to compare biologic monotherapy with a nonbiologic DMARD for the treatment of early RA patients with poor prognosis [31]. In this randomized controlled trial, 632 patients with early RA were followed for at least 1 year in a double-blind fashion. The patients included in this study had a mean disease duration of 12 months; had active RA with 10 or more swollen joints, 12 or more tender joints, an erythrocyte sedimentation rate greater than or equal to 28 mm, CRP greater than or equal to 2 mg/dL, or morning stiffness lasting 45 minutes or longer; and were at high risk for radiographic progression with positive rheumatoid factor or at least three erosions in hands or feet. Prior treatment with methotrexate was not allowed. Patients were randomized to receive either twice-weekly etanercept (10 mg or 25 mg) or weekly oral methotrexate (mean dose 19 mg/wk). After the blinded phase of the trial, 512 patients continued to receive the allocated treatment for an additional year in an open-label extension study [32].

Patients receiving etanercept showed more rapid clinical improvement compared with patients receiving methotrexate. During the 12 months of follow-up, patients receiving etanercept, 25 mg, had significantly better overall clinical response (area under the curve for ACR-N) compared with patients on methotrexate. The percentages of patients fulfilling ACR 20, ACR 50, and ACR 70 were significantly different between the methotrexate group and the etanercept, 25 mg, group during the first 6 months and comparable for all groups thereafter, although etanercept, 25 mg, was numerically superior to methotrexate. At 2 years of follow-up, the ACR 20 response was significantly higher in the etanercept, 25 mg, group than in the methotrexate group (72% versus 59%; $P = .005$). Progression of radiologic damage was significantly lower in the etanercept, 25 mg, group compared with the methotrexate group and the etanercept, 10 mg group. Of patients receiving methotrexate, 51% had no increase in total Sharp score (ΔSHS <0.5) compared with 63% of patients receiving 25 mg of etanercept ($P = .017$), and 58% compared with 70% had no increase in the erosion score ($P = 0.012$). After 1 year of follow-up, 55% of patients receiving methotrexate and patients receiving etanercept, 25 mg, showed a clinically relevant improvement in functional ability (ΔHAQ from baseline >0.5). At 2 years of follow-up, this percentage remained stable for the etanercept, 25 mg, group, whereas the percentage in the methotrexate group declined to 37% ($P<.001$). During the 2-year period, significantly more patients receiving methotrexate discontinued therapy because of adverse events (12% for methotrexate and 5% and 7% for etanercept, 10 mg and 25 mg).

After the follow-up phase of 2 years, patients were followed in an open-label fashion. Patients on etanercept, 10 mg or 25 mg, all continued with etanercept, 25 mg. In patients receiving methotrexate, etanercept, 25 mg, was added to methotrexate, or methotrexate was replaced by etanercept, 25 mg. At 3 years of follow-up, the patients who switched from methotrexate or etanercept, 10 mg, showed additional benefit of etanercept, 25 mg, with approximately equal percentages of patients fulfilling ACR 20 as in the patients who initially were allocated to etanercept, 25 mg (ACR 20 72%, 81%, and 76%). Observations at 3 and 4 years of follow-up showed sustained safety and clinically efficacy of treatment with etanercept, 25 mg [33,34].

The results of the ERA trial show that over 2 years of follow-up, etanercept, 25 mg, is superior to methotrexate in reduction of progression of joint damage and maintaining functional improvement in early, aggressive RA. This trial and the TEMPO trial underline the benefits of methotrexate as monotherapy, however, resulting in arrest of progression of joint damage in 51% (ERA) and 60% (TEMPO) of the patients. In the ERA trial, clinical improvement is more rapid with etanercept, but is comparable with methotrexate after the initial 6 months, and by switching to etanercept, 25 mg, after 2 years, equal clinical improvement can be achieved. Additional analyses need to determine whether the initial rapid clinical improvement results in ongoing lower progression of joint damage and sustained better physical function. Because an improvement in total SHS was observed in the patients on the combination in the TEMPO trial, the course of radiologic damage during long-term follow-up of the ERA-patients would be interesting.

Etanercept in early rheumatoid arthritis: relative benefits compared with established rheumatoid arthritis

That the initial phase may prove to be crucial in future functional ability is indicated by the results of the post-hoc analysis comparing functional improvement of early RA patients with that of patients with established RA, both receiving etanercept [35]. The early RA patients comprised the 207 patients participating in the ERA trial and randomized to receive etanercept, 25mg twice weekly. For the established RA group, 464 patients were derived from a cohort in which long-term safety of etanercept monotherapy was studied [36]. Before start of etanercept, this latter group of patients had had suboptimal responses with 1 or more DMARDs, including methotrexate. These patients were treated with either 10 mg or 25 mg of etanercept twice weekly, with 84% of all patients receiving 25 mg during the whole study period. At baseline, the patients with established RA had a higher mean disease duration of 12 years compared with

1 year for the ERA group, higher mean HAQ scores (1.64 versus 1.45; $P = .004$), and higher mean CRP levels (4.5 versus 3.3; $P = .005$), but were comparable with the ERA group for other baseline characteristics. HAQ scores during 3 years of follow-up were compared between the two groups with HAQ scores available for 3 years for 148 ERA patients (71%) and for 288 established RA patients (62%). In both groups, rapid, sustained clinical improvement was achieved with etanercept with percentages of patients achieving ACR 20, ACR 50, and ACR 70 responses at 3 years of 76%, 56%, and 33% in the ERA group compared with 77%, 50%, and 28% in the established RA group. Improvement of function also was rapid and sustained in both groups with more than 50% of patients already improved more than 0.2 points in HAQ (standing for clinically relevant improvement) at 2 weeks after start of etanercept. The magnitude of improvement was significantly greater, however, in patients with early RA. At 3 years of follow-up, more early RA patients had achieved clinically relevant functional improvement (85%) compared with patients with established RA (75%; $P = .0125$ corrected for baseline HAQ). An explanation for the observed difference in improvement of function may be the underlying existing joint damage in the patients with established RA, whereas in the ERA patients, joint inflammation is the main cause of functional impairment.

Although the analysis has obvious limitations—a post-hoc analysis on two populations from different studies with the patients with established RA already having failed on methotrexate—this study emphasizes that early intervention results in better functional improvement. Long-term follow-up of the progression of radiologic joint damage in both of these groups and in the different groups originally started in the ERA trial needs to clarify whether the initial rapid clinical improvement will turn out to be crucial in terms of future joint damage progression and further functional decline.

Adalimumab

Adalimumab (D2E7, Humira) is a fully human monoclonal TNF-α antibody with high specifity and affinity for TNF-α. It is structurally and functionally analogous to naturally occurring human IgG1 with a half-life of approximately 14 days, and it exerts its therapeutic effects by blocking the interaction between TNF-α and the TNF cell surface receptors. Adalimumab was developed for treatment of RA as monotherapy and in combination with methotrexate and is administered by subcutaneous injections. Currently, adalimumab is approved for treatment of RA as monotherapy [14,18].

The ARMADA trial (Anti-TNF Research Study Program of the Monoclonal Antibody Adalimumab in RA) evaluated the efficacy and safety of adalimumab in combination with methotrexate in patients with active RA despite methotrexate and with mean disease duration of 12.3 years [37]. All groups receiving methotrexate and adalimumab showed significant higher clinical response rates; adalimumab was well tolerated. Radiographic benefits of adalimumab added to continuing methotrexate therapy were investigated in a placebo-controlled study with 619 patients with mean disease duration of 10.9 years and previous incomplete responses to methotrexate [15]. The progression of radiologic joint damage was significantly lower in patients receiving adalimumab at 24 and 52 weeks. After 1 year, 62% and 58% of patients on adalimumab (40 mg every other week and 20 mg/week) compared with 46% of patients taking placebo had not developed new erosions.

The clinical efficacy and safety of adalimumab as monotherapy were evaluated in a 26-week, double-blind, placebo-controlled trial with 544 patients with long-standing severe RA despite treatment with at least one DMARD and mean disease duration of 11 years [38]. Treatment with adalimumab as monotherapy resulted in rapid and sustained clinical improvement, with more patients achieving ACR 20, ACR 50, and ACR 70 compared with placebo. Patients on adalimumab showed better functional improvement. The number of adverse events per total years of treatment was comparable between adalimumab and placebo, and serious infections were reported equally in both groups.

Adalimumab in early rheumatoid arthritis

The following results were published concerning the effectiveness and safety of adalimumab in early RA. The PREMIER study compared the combination of methotrexate (rapidly increased to 20 mg/w) and adalimumab (40 mg every other week) to either drug alone over 2 years [39]. A total of 799 methotrexate-naïve patients with active RA of less than 3 years' duration (mean duration 0.7 year) were included. Patients receiving the combination showed rapid, sustained clinical improvement with greater proportions of patients fulfilling ACR 20, ACR 50, and ACR 70 starting from week 2 during the entire 2-year study period with ACR 50 response at 1 year of 61%, 42%, and 46% and at 2 years of 59%, 37%, and 43% and with ACR 70 response at 1 year of 46%, 26%, and 28% and at 2 years of 47%, 27%, and 28% for the combination, adalimumab, and methotrexate (see Table 1). Of patients receiving the combination, 49% achieved a continuous ACR 70 response for 6 months or more compared with 25% and 27% for adalimumab and methotrexate alone.

More patients receiving the combination achieved remission (DAS 28 < 2.6): 50% for the combination compared with 25% for both monotherapy groups at 2 years of follow-up. Compared with patients receiving methotrexate monotherapy, patients receiving adalimumab had lower progression of total SHS with mean change of SHS over 2 years of 1.9, 5.5, and 10.4 for the combination, adalimumab alone, and methotrexate alone. There were no differences in frequencies of adverse effects among the three groups. This study shows the clinical and radiologic benefits of adalimumab and methotrexate in early RA compared with each drug alone with a remarkably high percentages of patients on the combination achieving remission (50%) and sustained ACR 70 (49%).

An open-label extension study evaluated the prevalence, sustainability, and clinical features of persistent remission in 846 patients with early or long-standing RA all treated with adalimumab, 40 mg every other week, and methotrexate [40]. The period in persistent remission was calculated from the first to the last visit continuously showing a DAS 28 less than 2.6 for 6 months or more with one DAS 28 2.6/y or greater allowed. A total of 29% of patients achieved clinical remission after a mean period of 10 months, and remission was sustained for a mean period of 25 months (range 6–56). Of patients with early RA (≤2 years) 31% achieved remission compared with 29% of patients with long-standing disease. Mean time to remission and mean duration of remission were comparable between patients with early and patients with longstanding RA. The 36 patients with early RA who achieved remission had a higher CRP and DAS 28 and longer duration of morning stiffness at baseline compared with the 209 patients with more long-standing RA (>2 years) who achieved remission. This finding suggests that the combination of methotrexate and adalimumab can have even more impact on disease course when applied early.

Safety considerations

Accompanying the great successes of the TNF-α inhibitors, there have been concerns about the safety profile. Because TNF-α is a key proinflammatory cytokine playing an important role in the host defense-system, it was reasoned that TNF-α blockade could lead to increased incidence of infections and malignancies in particular. Present-day knowledge is based mainly on long-term follow-up of clinical trials, postmarketing surveillance, and case reports and notably concerns patients with long-standing and refractory RA. Several issues have emerged from this follow-up, including injection site and infusion reactions, serious infections including tuberculosis, and lymphomas. Injection site and infusion reactions are mostly mild to moderate, are manageable, and rarely lead to discontinuation of therapy. Special consideration has to be made in the occurrence of problems including serious infections and tuberculosis. In the latter, a detailed evaluation for latent tuberculosis should be made before starting therapy. Careful monitoring is necessary to minimize the risk for other opportunistic and serious infections. In case of an infection, standard medical treatment generally is sufficient. TNF-α inhibitors should not be started or should be discontinued until the infection has been treated adequately. Data about the risk of developing lymphomas are difficult to interpret because the incidence of lymphomas is increased in RA [41]. Treatment with TNF-α inhibitors is associated with increased standardized incidence ratios for lymphomas, but the differences between various treatment groups are very little. Part of the difference may be due to the application of TNF-α inhibitors preferentially in patients with long-standing and severe RA who might have a higher risk to develop lymphomas in general.

Other issues related to the TNF-α inhibitors, such as autoimmune disorders, cardiac insufficiency, demyelinating diseases, and interstitial lung disease also may need to be considered even though data for these are weak. If the patients are informed about the various safety aspects and outcomes, the risk-to-benefit ratio for treatment with TNF-α inhibitors remains favorable. Long-term follow-up of various groups of RA patients needs to elucidate whether the risk-to-benefit ratio of patients with early RA is comparable to patients with established disease [41–43].

Therapeutic strategy in early rheumatoid arthritis

The Aspire study, the TEMPO trial, and the PREMIER study all independently showed the superiority of the combination of methotrexate and biologic in early and in long-standing RA. Each of these studies also emphasized the effectiveness of methotrexate and biologic monotherapy, however, and left unanswered which treatment strategy should be employed in patients presenting with RA. Should therapy be started with one DMARD, which, if unsuccessful, would be replaced with another DMARD or with a TNF-α inhibitor? Or should treatment be aggressive from the beginning with a combination of proven DMARDs or with a combination including a TNF-α inhibitor?

To find out which strategy would yield the best outcome, a head-to-head comparison of four aggressive treatment strategies in patients with early, DMARD-naïve RA was made, the BeSt study [44]. This randomized, single-blinded clinical trial compared sequential monotherapy, step-up combination therapy, initial combination therapy, and initial biologic therapy for functional ability and radiographic damage. The common goal in all strategies was to reduce disease activity rapidly and persistently by tight monitoring and immediate adjustment of therapy in case of an insufficient response (DAS >2.4). If the clinical response was consistently adequate (DAS ≤2.4 for at least 6 months), medication was tapered until only one drug remained. A total of 508 patients were included with median symptom duration of 23 weeks and with active RA (six or more swollen and six or more tender joints, erythrocyte sedimentation rate ≥28 mm/hr, or visual analog scale global health ≥20 mm). After 2 years, 42% of patients in all groups were in clinical remission (DAS <1.6), showing that very low disease activity is an achievable goal with aggressive strategies. Over 2 years of follow-up, cumulative disease activity and cumulative functional impairment were lower in the initial combination group and the initial biologic group. These latter groups especially showed a more rapid improvement of DAS and HAQ during the first 3 months. At 1 and 2 years, mean DAS was equal for all four groups, and mean HAQ was only significantly higher in the sequential monotherapy group compared with the initial combination and the initial biologic groups. Progression of radiologic joint damage was significantly lower for the groups starting with a combination or a biologic, although the differences were small with median ΔSHS of 2 for sequential monotherapy and step-up and 1 for the groups with initial combination or a biologic. The number of adverse events was equal for all groups.

Data for the number of treatment switches varied among the four groups with in general fewer adjustments in the groups starting with a combination or a biologic. In the group with sequential monotherapy, in which in sequential order therapy could be switched from methotrexate to sulfasalazine to leflunomide to methotrexate plus infliximab, 33% of patients still received methotrexate at the end of the second year. Consequently, in approximately one third of patients with early RA, a low disease activity could be maintained with methotrexate monotherapy. In the group with the biologic, patients started with methotrexate, 25 mg/wk, plus infliximab, 3 mg/kg at 0, 2, and 6 weeks and every 8 weeks thereafter. Disease activity was assessed before each infliximab infusion. If the DAS was greater than 2.4, the infliximab dose was increased to 6, 7.5, and 10 mg/kg, and finally patients were switched to sulfasalazine. In case of consistently adequate response, infliximab was tapered and finally discontinued, and next methotrexate was tapered to 10 mg/wk. Of all patients who started with methotrexate and infliximab, 72% remained in the initial treatment step. During the 2-year study period, infliximab could be discontinued after an average of 1 year without disease flare in 54% of the patients, and methotrexate afterward could be tapered to a mean dose of 12.2 mg/wk. SHS progression was observed less frequently in responders compared with patients who failed on treatment with increasing dosages of infliximab. In summary, after 2 years of follow-up, 33% of patients in group 1 compared with 54% of patients in group 4 were receiving methotrexate monotherapy.

All patients participating in the BeSt study were asked whether their general health was improved with treatment. Overall the results were positive with optimal results in the biologic group, in which 91% of patients stated that their general health had improved by therapy. This group was followed in descending order by sequential monotherapy (87%), step-up (85%), and combination therapy (77%).

Summary

Trials such as TEMPO, Aspire, BeSt, and PREMIER all show that treatment with a TNF-α inhibitor, infliximab, etanercept, or adalimumab, especially in combination with methotrexate is a step forward in treatment of early RA. Long-term follow-up of patients treated early with a biologic has to clarify certain issues, however, as listed in Box 1:

Additional observations and long-term follow-up on the use of biologics in various groups of patients need to point out the exact balance in terms of cost and benefit for the individual patient with early RA. Overall, the promising results of the trials discussed in this article indicate that the treatment paradigm for RA has been shifted toward using TNF-α inhibitors. By defining high treatment goals and by the use of aggressive treatment strategies, the best outcome is obtained, and remission or low disease activity becomes an achievable goal for a greater

---

Box 1. Issues in long-term follow-up of patients treated early with biologics

- *Timing:* Whether the impact of the combination biologic and methotrexate applied during the early stages of RA (window of opportunity) will turn out to be crucial for long-term joint damage progression needs to be clarified.
- *Costs:* Because biologics currently are far more expensive than the traditional DMARDs, data concerning absenteeism and additional use of health-care services are important.
- *Disease severity:* Biologics have proven to work well in severe, active RA, but might work even better in moderate disease.
- *Safety:* Current knowledge is based mainly on long-term follow-up in patients with long-standing RA; long-term follow-up of early RA-patients needs to clarify the risk profile for these patients.
- *Other biologics:* Apart from the TNF-α inhibitors, anakinra and a variety of other agents have been developed and are currently under investigation.

---

proportion of patients. Success or failure of treatment should be evaluated regularly as part of everyday practice. Because current data show that TNF-α plays a key role in disease progression, TNF-α inhibitors should be considered for use as soon as traditional therapies do not result in the desired treatment goal. When severe joint damage has developed, TNF-α inhibitors can improve disease status significantly. If there is no severe, irreversible destruction, the use of TNF-α inhibitors would have a greater impact on functional ability by preservation of the joints.

References

[1] Pincus T, Callahan LF, Sale WG, et al. Severe functional declines, work disability, and increased mortality in seventy-five rheumatoid arthritis patients studied over nine years. Arthritis Rheum 1984;27:864–72.

[2] Wolfe F, Mitchell DM, Sibley JT, et al. The mortality of rheumatoid arthritis. Arthritis Rheum 1994;37:481–94.

[3] Wolfe F. The natural history of rheumatoid arthritis. J Rheumatol Suppl 1996;44:13–22.

[4] Mottonen TT. Prediction of erosiveness and rate of development of new erosions in early rheumatoid arthritis. Ann Rheum Dis 1988;47:648–53.

[5] Boers M, Verhoeven AC, Markusse HM, et al. Randomised comparison of combined step-down prednisolone, methotrexate and sulphasalazine with sulphasalazine alone in early rheumatoid arthritis. Lancet 1997;350:309–18.

[6] Lard LR, Visser H, Speyer I, et al. Early versus delayed treatment in patients with recent-onset

rheumatoid arthritis: comparison of two cohorts who received different treatment strategies. Am J Med 2001;111:446–51.

[7] van Jaarsveld CH, Jacobs JW, van der Veen MJ, et al. Aggressive treatment in early rheumatoid arthritis: a randomised controlled trial. On behalf of the Rheumatic Research Foundation Utrecht, The Netherlands. Ann Rheum Dis 2000;59:468–77.

[8] van der Heide A, Jacobs JW, Bijlsma JW, et al. The effectiveness of early treatment with "second-line" antirheumatic drugs: a randomized, controlled trial. Ann Intern Med 1996;124: 699–707.

[9] Egsmose C, Lund B, Borg G, et al. Patients with rheumatoid arthritis benefit from early 2nd line therapy: 5 year followup of a prospective double blind placebo controlled study. J Rheumatol 1995;22:2208–13.

[10] Korpela M, Laasonen L, Hannonen P, et al. Retardation of joint damage in patients with early rheumatoid arthritis by initial aggressive treatment with disease-modifying antirheumatic drugs: five-year experience from the FIN-RACo study. Arthritis Rheum 2004;50:2072–81.

[11] Landewe RB, Boers M, Verhoeven AC, et al. COBRA combination therapy in patients with early rheumatoid arthritis: long-term structural benefits of a brief intervention. Arthritis Rheum 2002; 46:347–56.

[12] Verstappen SM, Jacobs JW, Bijlsma JW, et al. Five-year followup of rheumatoid arthritis patients after early treatment with disease-modifying antirheumatic drugs versus treatment according to the pyramid approach in the first year. Arthritis Rheum 2003;48:1797–807.

[13] Grigor C, Capell H, Stirling A, et al. Effect of a treatment strategy of tight control for rheumatoid arthritis (the TICORA study): a single-blind randomised controlled trial. Lancet 2004; 364:263–9.

[14] Shanahan JC, Moreland LW, Carter RH. Upcoming biologic agents for the treatment of rheumatic diseases. Curr Opin Rheumatol 2003;15:226–36.

[15] Keystone EC, Kavanaugh AF, Sharp JT, et al. Radiographic, clinical, and functional outcomes of treatment with adalimumab (a human anti-tumor necrosis factor monoclonal antibody) in patients with active rheumatoid arthritis receiving concomitant methotrexate therapy: a randomized, placebo-controlled, 52-week trial. Arthritis Rheum 2004;50:1400–11.

[16] Lipsky PE, van der Heijde DM, St Clair EW, et al. Infliximab and methotrexate in the treatment of rheumatoid arthritis. Anti-Tumor Necrosis Factor Trial in Rheumatoid Arthritis with Concomitant Therapy Study Group. N Engl J Med 2000;343:1594–602.

[17] Klareskog L, van der Heijde D, de Jager JP, et al. Therapeutic effect of the combination of etanercept and methotrexate compared with each treatment alone in patients with rheumatoid arthritis: double-blind randomised controlled trial. Lancet 2004;363:675–81.

[18] Furst DE, Breedveld FC, Kalden JR, et al. Updated consensus statement on biological agents, specifically tumour necrosis factor alpha (TNFalpha) blocking agents and interleukin-1 receptor antagonist (IL-1ra), for the treatment of rheumatic diseases, 2004. Ann Rheum Dis 2004; 63(Suppl):ii2–12.

[19] Elliott MJ, Maini RN, Feldmann M, et al. Randomised double-blind comparison of chimeric monoclonal antibody to tumour necrosis factor alpha (cA2) versus placebo in rheumatoid arthritis. Lancet 1994;344:1105–10.

[20] Maini R, St Clair EW, Breedveld F, et al. Infliximab (chimeric anti-tumour necrosis factor alpha monoclonal antibody) versus placebo in rheumatoid arthritis patients receiving concomitant methotrexate: a randomised phase III trial. ATTRACT Study Group. Lancet 1999; 354:1932–9.

[21] Maini RN, Breedveld FC, Kalden JR, et al. Sustained improvement over two years in physical function, structural damage, and signs and symptoms among patients with rheumatoid arthritis treated with infliximab and methotrexate. Arthritis Rheum 2004;50:1051–65.

[22] Breedveld FC, Emery P, Keystone E, et al. Infliximab in active early rheumatoid arthritis. Ann Rheum Dis 2004;63:149–55.

[23] St Clair EW, van der Heijde DM, Smolen JS, et al. Combination of infliximab and methotrexate therapy for early rheumatoid arthritis: a randomized, controlled trial. Arthritis Rheum 2004; 50:3432–43.

[24] Taylor PC, Steuer A, Gruber J, et al. Comparison of ultrasonographic assessment of synovitis and joint vascularity with radiographic evaluation in a randomized, placebo-controlled study of infliximab therapy in early rheumatoid arthritis. Arthritis Rheum 2004;50:1107–16.

[25] Conaghan PG, Quinn MA, O'Connor P, et al. Can very high-dose anti-tumor necrosis factor blockade at onset of rheumatoid arthritis produce long-term remission? Arthritis Rheum 2002; 46:1971–2.

[26] Quinn MA, Conaghan PG, O'Connor PJ, et al. Very early treatment with infliximab in addition to methotrexate in early, poor-prognosis rheumatoid arthritis reduces magnetic resonance imaging evidence of synovitis and damage, with sustained benefit after infliximab withdrawal: results from a twelve-month randomized, double-blind, placebo-controlled trial. Arthritis Rheum 2005;52:27–35.

[27] Moreland LW, Baumgartner SW, Schiff MH, et al. Treatment of rheumatoid arthritis with a recombinant human tumor necrosis factor receptor (p75)-Fc fusion protein. N Engl J Med 1997; 337:141–7.

[28] Kremer JM, Weinblatt ME, Bankhurst AD, et al. Etanercept added to background methotrexate therapy in patients with rheumatoid arthritis: continued observations. Arthritis Rheum 2003;48: 1493–9.

[29] Van der Heijde D, Klareskog L, Wajdula J, et al for the TEMPO study investigators. Halting of radiographic progression in RA patients treated with etanercept and methotrexate; year 2 results from the TEMPO trial. Arthritis Rheum 2004;50:4098.

[30] Klareskog L, Van der Heijde D, Wajdula J, et al for the TEMPO study investigators. Therapeutic response following two years of treatment with etanercept, methotrexate, or combination therapy in patients with early rheumatoid arthritis (RA). Arthritis Rheum 2004;50:s238.

[31] Bathon JM, Martin RW, Fleischmann RM, et al. A comparison of etanercept and methotrexate in patients with early rheumatoid arthritis. N Engl J Med 2000;343:1586–93.

[32] Genovese MC, Bathon JM, Martin RW, et al. Etanercept versus methotrexate in patients with early rheumatoid arthritis: two-year radiographic and clinical outcomes. Arthritis Rheum 2002; 46:1443–50.

[33] Genovese MC, Martin RW, Fleischmann RM, et al. Etanercept (Enbrel) in early erosive rheumatoid arthritis (ERA trial): observations at 3 years. Arthritis Rheum 2001;44:s78.

[34] Genovese MC, Martin RW, Fleischmann RM, et al. Etanercept (Enbrel) in early erosive rhuematoid atrrthritis (ERA Trial): observations at 4 years. Arthritis Rheum 2002; 46:s530.

[35] Baumgartner SW, Fleischmann RM, Moreland LW, et al. Etanercept (Enbrel) in patients with rheumatoid arthritis with recent onset versus established disease: improvement in disability. J Rheumatol 2004;31:1532–7.

[36] Moreland LW, Cohen SB, Baumgartner SW, et al. Long-term safety and efficacy of etanercept in patients with rheumatoid arthritis. J Rheumatol 2001;28:1238–44.

[37] Weinblatt ME, Keystone EC, Furst DE, et al. Adalimumab, a fully human anti-tumor necrosis factor alpha monoclonal antibody, for the treatment of rheumatoid arthritis in patients taking concomitant methotrexate: the ARMADA trial. Arthritis Rheum 2003;48:35–45.

[38] van de Putte LB, Atkins C, Malaise M, et al. Efficacy and safety of adalimumab as monotherapy in patients with rheumatoid arthritis for whom previous disease modifying antirheumatic drug treatment has failed. Ann Rheum Dis 2004;63:508–16.

[39] Breedveld FC, Kavanaugh AF, Cohen SB, et al. Early treatment of rheumatoid arthritis (RA) with adalimumab (HUMIRA) plus methotrexate vs. adalimumab alone or methotrexate alone: the Premier study. Arthritis Rheum 2004;50:4096.

[40] Emery P, Kalden JR, Spencer-Green GT, Segurado OG. Adalimumab (HUMIRA) plus methotrexate induces sustained remission in both early and long- standing rheumatoid arthritis. Arthritis Rheum 2004;50:S183.

[41] Wolfe F, Michaud K. Lymphoma in rheumatoid arthritis: the effect of methotrexate and anti-tumor necrosis factor therapy in 18,572 patients. Arthritis Rheum 2004;50:1740–51.

[42] Kavanaugh A, Keystone EC. The safety of biologic agents in early rheumatoid arthritis. Exp Rheumatol 2003;21(Suppl 31):s203–8.

[43] Fleischmann R, Yocum D. Does safety make a difference in selecting the right TNF antagonist? Arthritis Res Ther 2004;6(Suppl):8.

[44] Goekoop-Ruiterman YPM, De Vries-Bouwstra JK, Van Zeben D, et al. Treatment strategies in early rheumatoid arthritis: clinical and radiological outcomes after 2 year follow-up of the BeSt study. Arthritis Rheum 2004;50:4096.

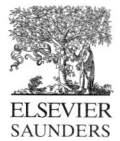
ELSEVIER
SAUNDERS

RHEUMATIC
DISEASE CLINICS
OF NORTH AMERICA

Rheum Dis Clin N Am 31 (2005) 763–772

Potential for Altering Rheumatoid Arthritis Outcome

Mark A. Quinn, MBChB, MRCP[a], Paul Emery, MA, MD, FRCP[a,b,*]

[a]Academic Unit of Musculoskeletal Disease, Department of Rheumatology,
Chapel Allerton Hospital, Leeds, UK
[b]Leeds Teaching Hospitals Trust, Chapel Allerton Hospital, Leeds, UK

The potential for disproportionately altering outcome in the early stages of rheumatoid arthritis (RA) was first hypothesized in the early 1990s [1]. This window of opportunity hypothesis for therapeutic intervention in RA is based on the existence of a time frame within which there is a potential for a greater response to therapy, resulting in sustained benefits or, perhaps most important, a chance of cure. Given the persistent, progressive, damaging, inflammatory nature of RA, this approach to altering outcome in the early stages seems attractive.

Inflammation is now the therapeutic target

Until the 1990s, the conventional approach to treatment of RA had been a protocol that started with the least toxic and least effective therapies (eg, analgesics and nonsteroidal anti-inflammatory drugs [NSAIDs]), followed by more effective, but what were thought to be more toxic drugs (eg, corticosteroids and disease-modifying antirheumatic drugs [DMARDs]); this was the classic treatment pyramid. It was common practice that DMARDs were initiated only when patients had demonstrable radiologic damage and so had justified their treatment. In 1985, rheumatology textbooks still were recommending 2 years of NSAIDs before starting DMARDs [2]. This treatment approach was based on the notion

* Corresponding author. Academic Unit of Musculoskeletal Disease Department of Rheumatology, Chapel Allerton Hospital, 2nd Floor, Chapel Town Road, Leeds LS7 4SA, UK.
E-mail address: p.emery@leeds.ac.uk (P. Emery).

0889-857X/05/$ – see front matter © 2005 Elsevier Inc. All rights reserved.
doi:10.1016/j.rdc.2005.07.008
rheumatic.theclinics.com

that RA in general was mild, with joint damage and disability occurring slowly. The earliest RA cohort studies disproved this belief, however, with most patients experiencing significant disability and mortality after long-term follow-up [3–5]. These data changed rheumatologists' perceptions of outcomes in RA and altered approaches to therapy. Later radiologic outcome studies showed that damage occurred earlier in disease than was initially thought with 90% of patients having radiologic evidence of damage by the end of 2 years of symptoms [6]. More recent studies using modern imaging techniques, such as MRI and ultrasonography, have confirmed evidence of damage within weeks of onset of symptoms [7,8]. MRI lesions have been shown to correlate reliably with later radiographic erosions [9] with a mean lag time of approximately 2 years [10]. Damage occurs earlier than was first thought, and waiting for evidence of radiographic damage before intervention no longer can be reasonably justified.

In addition to increasing evidence of damage and disability in RA, there was the growing evidence of the relationship of these with inflammation. C-reactive protein (CRP) is regarded as a surrogate marker of inflammation, and there is now a plethora of data in the literature relating high levels of CRP to radiographic [11–13] and functional [14] outcomes and localized and systemic bone density loss [15–17]. These data becomes more clinically relevant when time-integrated values for CRP are considered [18]. Despite these data, it has been suggested that damage may occur in the face of control of inflammatory disease [19]. Imaging has helped elucidate the relationship of inflammatory disease with bone damage. MRI studies have shown a direct correlation between synovial volume and erosive changes [20] and evidence of a threshold effect, below which damage does not occur. These findings concur with data whereby damage occurs only in clinically affected joints [21]. From these data, there seems to be no dissociation of inflammatory disease with radiographic damage, and synovitis should be the primary therapeutic target. There has been a shift in thinking since the 1990s, with a switch in the therapeutic target from treating the erosion-to-erosion prevention through suppression of inflammation.

Early therapy is effective

There is a body of evidence from therapeutic studies in early RA to support the early use of DMARD therapy. Most studies show a quantitative benefit in clinical outcome and show delayed introduction of DMARD therapy to be detrimental. There is some evidence to suggest the best predictor of response to therapy is symptom duration. Anderson and colleagues [22] showed in an analysis of 1435 patients from 11 different studies that disease duration was of foremost importance in predicting response to DMARD therapy. Of patients presenting with less than 1 year's disease duration, 53% showed a response, whereas later groups (1–2 years, 2–5 years, 5–10 years, and >10 years) showed diminished response with disease duration measured by American College of Rheumatology criteria (ACR 20). The opportunity for functicnal improvement also may be lost with delayed introduction of therapy. In a study of 440 patients, patients treated early (<2 years) showed a significant improvement in function, measured by the Health Assessment Questionnaire, whereas patients with a longer disease duration showed little reversibility of their impairment [23]. Similarly, when early treatment was compared with delayed therapy after 8 months with oral gold, clinical benefit and sustained radiologic improvement were shown after 5 years' follow-up [24]. Van der Heide and colleagues [25] compared DMARD treatment with NSAIDs alone and delayed introduction of DMARDs. All clinically relevant variables were improved at 1 year. No significant difference was detected in radiographic progression; this may have been due to a significantly greater number of non–DMARD-treated patients discontinuing therapy, a greater use of intra-articular corticosteroid in the non-DMARD group, or a type-2 statistical error [25]. Other studies looking at any DMARD use versus NSAIDs or no therapy strongly favor DMARD use with respect to long-term disability index [26] and deformed or damaged joint and radiographic score [27]. In considering qualitative rather than quantitative improvement in outcome, fewer data are available. In a study of 448 RA patients, patients who presented with less than 5 years' disease duration maintained a lower mortality ratio over 21.5 years of follow-up compared with late presenters [28]. Early introduction of therapy seems the most effective therapeutic approach, but the debate continues with regard to whether this is a true alteration of pathologic process or simply a case of debulking inflammatory disease.

Can the outcome of rheumatoid arthritis be altered?

Searching for evidence to support alteration of disease process, many studies can be highlighted, and each offers an alternative approach and interpretation of efficacy.

Very early intervention may produce a qualitative difference in outcome

Green and colleagues [29] studied 63 patients with mild early inflammatory arthritis, defined as synovitis in two or more joints with less than 12 months of symptoms, longitudinally for 6 months. Mild disease was defined as one of the following: (1) duration of symptoms less than 3 months regardless of pattern of disease, (2) asymmetric disease, or (3) symmetric metacarpophalangeal joint disease, but with a low prognostic severity score based on predictors of poor outcome in terms of function and radiographic damage. The aims of the study were to determine the factors that predict persistence of inflammation 6 months after corticosteroid therapy and to assess the ability of the ACR criteria to select these patients. There was sufficient uncertainty about the outlook of these patients that a temporary delay in DMARD therapy was believed to be ethical. The initial treatment was with a single dose of corticosteroids given intramuscularly (120 mg of methylprednisolone or 80 mg if patient weighed < 60 kg) or intra-articularly in cases with fewer than four affected joints. The factors associated with outcome at 6 months subsequently were examined. In this group, the best predictor of persistence was disease duration 12 weeks or longer. With disease duration less than 12 weeks, the chance of remission was increased fivefold in patients satisfying the ACR RA criteria (Fig. 1). In analyzing the seronegative group for rheumatoid factor separately, patients in possession of the shared epitope were significantly more likely to have persistent disease. This finding suggests that in the rheumatoid factor–negative subgroup, the shared epitope may be of greater value. It already has been suggested that the shared epitope is associated with persistence rather than induction of arthritis [30]. No patients who were rheumatoid factor–positive and shared epitope–positive entered remission. After 12 weeks, classic features of RA were more predictive, with all but one patient with symmetric metacarpophalangeal synovitis having persistent disease. There was a trend for patients with a high CRP with very early disease to enter remission. Greater than 50% patients entered remission with a single dose of corticosteroid. ACR classification criteria were not predictive of persistence, and duration of symptoms alone was the best predictor of outcome. If these patients are considered to be RA patients in evolution, this may be preliminary evidence to suggest that intervention at this very early stage truly alters the disease process.

Mottenen and colleagues [31] studied the impact of the delay from the onset of symptoms to institution of DMARD therapy on remission rates in 195 patients with RA. In this further analysis of the FIN-RACo cohort, only disease duration significantly predicted remission rates in the monotherapy arm using a cutoff of 4 months' symptom duration ($P = .01$). No other recognized prognostic variable emerged in the logistic regression model. Perhaps also of interest here is that symptom duration did not predict remission in the combination therapy arm, suggesting aggressive therapy may abolish the impact of conventional prognostic

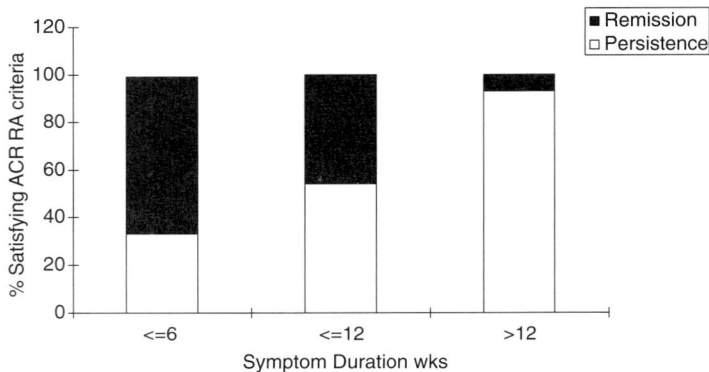

Fig. 1. Proportion of patients that satisfied ACR RA classification criteria [38] entering remission after a single corticosteroid challenge according to symptom duration.

factors. Lard and colleagues [32] reported similar findings in that the prognostic impact of the shared epitope was abolished in the aggressive arm in the COBRA study. These data suggest that disease duration could be pivotal in the therapeutic decision-making process when assessing a patient with early inflammatory arthritis.

Early combination disease-modifying antirheumatic drug therapy with corticosteroids produces long-lasting benefit

The ultimate aim of therapy is remission. In attempting remission induction, the COBRA study group reported a step-down therapeutic approach of sulfasalazine plus methotrexate plus prednisolone versus sulfasalazine alone [33]. Significant radiographic benefits were seen at 30 weeks, yet disease activity was comparable in the two groups after the steroid therapy was stopped. A follow-up study analyzing rate of radiographic progression between groups over the subsequent 4 to 5 years after the initial 56-week study period showed a reduction in radiographic progression rate in the combination therapy arm [34]. The findings are significant because of the sustained apparent benefit from 6 months of early aggressive therapy. This benefit may be simply a debulking effect, but such a long-term benefit is suggestive of an alteration or downgrading of the disease process.

Early biologic intervention in poor-prognosis early rheumatoid arthritis produces lasting benefits

A placebo-controlled pilot study in poor-prognosis early RA using infliximab and methotrexate versus methotrexate alone showed significant differences in functional outcome, quality of life, and MRI erosion scores at 12 months [35]. There were significant differences in the ACR responses at 12 months (ACR 50 70% versus 30%). After withdrawal of study drug (either infliximab or placebo) at 12 months and a further 12 months of observation, no patient showing response to infliximab had a flare of their disease requiring additional DMARD therapy, and median disease activity score (DAS 28) was maintained at remission levels (Fig. 2). In this study, not only was structural damage improved, but also disease activity benefits were seen early and were sustained, not only at 12 months, but also at 2 years. Even more important, functional and quality-of-life differences were attained very early and remained at 2 years' follow-up (Fig. 3); this was achieved without continued infliximab therapy. This study using infliximab as induction therapy has shown that early use of anti–tumor necrosis factor (TNF)-α can produce a sustained benefit in the most important subjective disease parameters of functional status and quality of life. This study differs from the studies of conventional DMARDs, in which structural damage is prevented, but patient-based assessments are not improved.

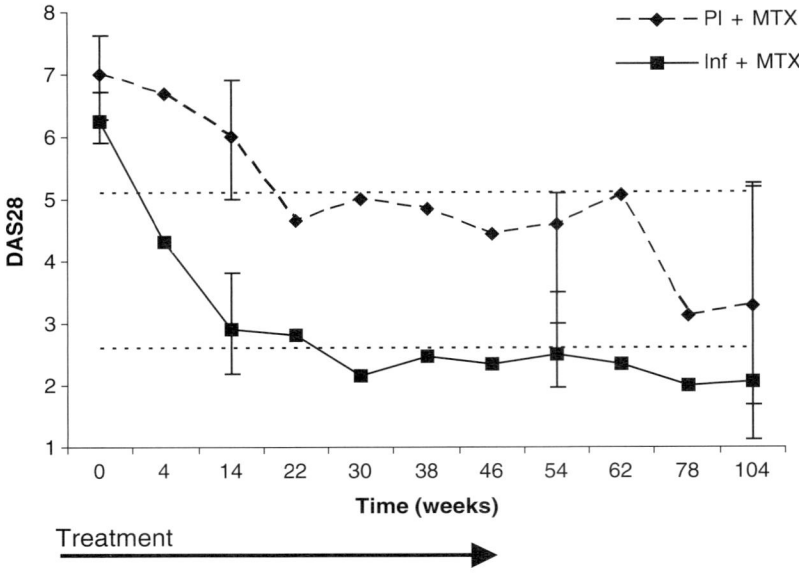

Fig. 2. Changes in median DAS 28 scores over time in patients treated with early infliximab (Inf) and methotrexate (MTX) compared with placebo (Pl) and MTX. Error bars = interquartile range.

Other studies using anti–TNF-α therapies in early RA also have shown clinical and radiographic benefits with continued use over 12 months. In the ASPIRE study, clinical improvements measured using ACR 20, ACR 50, and ACR 70, clinically significant improvements in Health Assessment Questionnaire and change in modified Sharp score all were significantly better with either of the infliximab and methotrexate arms (3 mg/kg and 6 mg/kg) compared with methotrexate alone [36]. In the PREMIER study, adalimumab and methotrexate in combination was superior to either of the drugs alone in terms of clinical improvement measured using ACR 50 and ACR 70, DAS 28 remission rates, and radiographic progression measured using total Sharp score over 2 years [37]. The combination arm achieved DAS 28 remission rates of 50%, the highest remission rates reported in RA studies. The long-term observation of these cohorts will add to current knowledge of early suppression of inflammatory disease in RA.

Long-term benefit from continued biologic therapy in early disease

In the Enbrel ERA study, 632 patients with early, active RA were randomized to receive either twice-weekly etanercept (10 mg or 25 mg) or weekly oral methotrexate (mean dose 19 mg/wk) for 1 year in a double-blind manner. Thereafter, 512 patients continued to receive randomized therapy (open-label) for a further year. The 12-month study showed rapid disease activity control with etanercept, which converged between groups by the 12-month time point [38]. At

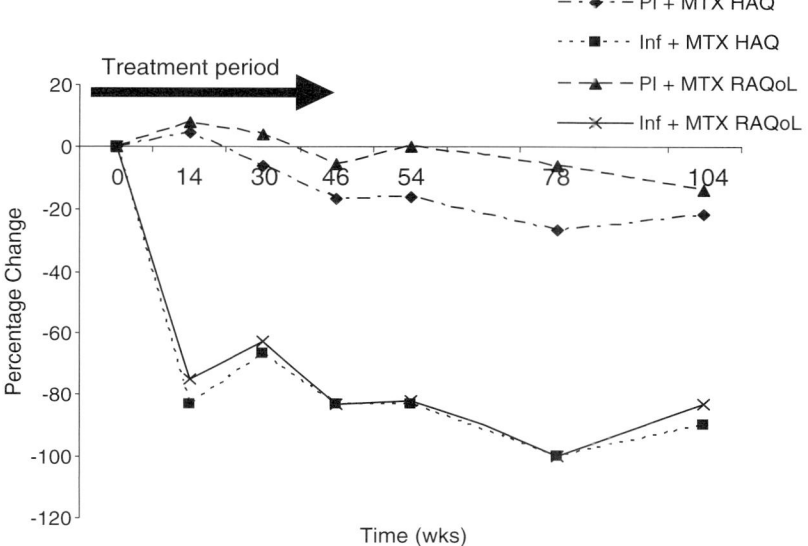

Fig. 3. Percentage change in median functional and quality-of-life scores over time in poor-prognosis early RA. HAQ, Health Assessment Questionnaire; Inf, infliximab; MTX, methotrexate; Pl, placebo; RAQoL, RA quality-of-life questionnaire.

12 months, there was a significant difference in Sharp erosion score in favor of the 25-mg etanercept group, but not for total score or joint space narrowing. With 12 months further follow-up, significant benefits were shown in total Sharp and erosion scores and functional improvement [39]. A greater number of patients achieved ACR 20 response in the 25-mg etanercept group at 24 months. Here benefits are seen in the second year after rapid and sustained suppression of disease activity with continued therapy, suggesting an important role of early suppression of inflammatory disease. This therapeutic benefit was seen only with continued use of etanercept, however. If it is assumed that etanercept is a better therapy than methotrexate alone, the increasingly significant benefits that were seen were due to an incremental effect over time.

New therapies alter expected outcomes in established rheumatoid arthritis

Klareskog and colleagues [40] showed high remission rates in patients with severe established RA using the combination of etanercept and methotrexate in the TEMPO study. Patients had mean disease duration of 6.8 years, 76% rheumatoid factor positive, mean Sharp erosion score at baseline of 9.5, and failed at least one prior DMARD. Traditionally, such patients would have fallen into a poor-prognosis group, yet with combination therapy using etanercept and methotrexate, DAS remission rates of 35% at 1 year [40] and 41% at 2 years were achieved [41]. Such results suggest that even in more established disease, good results are still possible with better treatments now available.

Summary

Previously, it was thought that more aggressive treatment regimens, usually combination therapies with corticosteroids, reduced damage for the duration of suppression of inflammation, and when these regimens were stopped, disease returned to previous levels. Long-term data now available with combination strategies and early data using infliximab suggest, however, there is evidence for a qualitative change in disease outcomes and perhaps disease mechanisms. Initial aggressive regimens result in debulking of inflammatory disease with improvement in damage and early outcome, and although the disease process continues, it seems attenuated subsequently.

Introducing conventional therapies within months of onset of disease would seem to offer the greatest opportunity for achieving remission and highlights the importance of early assessment in intervention in RA. After the first few months, aggressive therapeutic strategies would seem to be required to attain optimal outcomes. The place of therapies that inhibit TNF-α as initial therapy for RA cannot be fully supported yet, but data suggest an opportunity to make a difference exists with a limited duration of therapy at disease onset. Beyond the early phases, these therapies may be potent enough in a proportion of cases to rescue failing patients and reset the disease process.

The pathologic mechanisms to explain these data are not fully understood, but raise the question of a therapeutic window that may be exploited to gain maximum effect of therapy. A very early window of opportunity may exist (<16 weeks symptoms) in which early intervention may alter the propensity to persistence and offer the opportunity of cure. This time frame may be lengthened with the availability of more potent agents, such as the TNF-α antagonists. The success of therapy may depend on the ability to suppress inflammation completely. This ability depends on (1) the level of synovitis (proportional to and determined by disease duration) and (2) potency and duration of effective therapy. These avenues require further research to understand fully the pathologic processes behind these findings, but the evidence for a therapeutic window of opportunity continues to develop.

References

[1] Emery P. Prognosis in inflammatory arthritis: the value of HLA genotyping and oncological analogy. The Dunlop Dotteridge Lecture. J Rheumatol 1997;24:1436–42.

[2] Lightfoot Jr RW. Treatment of rheumatoid arthritis. In: McCarty DJ, editor. Arthritis and allied conditions. Philadelphia: Lea & Febiger; 1985. p. 668–76.

[3] Scott DL, Symmons DP, Coulton BL, et al. Long term outcome of treating rheumatoid arthritis: results after 20 years. Lancet 1987;1(8542):1108–11.

[4] Pincus T, Callahan LF, Sale WG, et al. Severe functional declines, work disbaility and increased mortality in seventy-five rheumatoid arthritis patients studied over nine years. Arthritis Rheum 1984;27:864–72.

[5] Rasker JJ, Cosh JA. The natural history of rheumatoid arthritis: a fifteen year follow up study: the prognostic significance of features noted in the first year. Clin Rheumatol 1984;3:11–20.

[6] Emery P. The optimal management of early rheumatoid disease: the key to preventing disability. Br J Rheumatol 1994;33:765–8.

[7] McGonagle D, Conaghan PG, O'Connor P, et al. The relationship between synovitis and bone changes in early untreated rheumatoid arthritis Arthritis Rheum 1999;42:1706–11.

[8] Wakefield RJ, Gibbon WW, Conaghan PG, et al. The value of sonography in the detection of bone erosions in patients with rheumatoid arthritis: a comparison with conventional radiography. Arthritis Rheum 2000;43:2762–70.

[9] McQueen FM, Benton N, Crabbe J, et al. What is the fate of erosions in early rheumatoid arthritis? Tracking individual lesions using x rays and magnetic resonance imaging over the first two years of disease. Ann Rheum Dis 2001;60:859–68.

[10] Østergaard M, Hansen M, Stoltenberg M, et al. New radiographic bone erosions in the wrists of patients with rheumatoid arthritis are detectable with magnetic resonance imaging a median of two years earlier. Arthritis Rheum 2003;48:2128–31.

[11] Van Leeuwen MA, Van Rijswijk MH, Sluiter WJ, et al. Individual relationship between progression of radiological damage and the acute phase response in early rheumatoid arthritis: towards development of a decision support system. J Rheumatol 1997;24:20–7.

[12] Fex E, Eberhardt K, Saxne T. Tissue derived macromolecules and markers of inflammation in serum in early rheumatoid arthritis: relationship to development of joint destruction in hands and feet. Br J Rheumatol 1997;36:1161–5.

[13] Amos RA, Constable TJ, Crockson RA, et al. Rheumatoid arthritis: relationship of C-reactive protein and erythrocyte sedimentation rates and radiographic change. BMJ 1977;1:195–7.

[14] Devlin J, Gough A, Huissoon A, et al. The acute phase and function in early RA: CRP levels correlate with functional outcome. J Rheumatol 1997;24:9–13.

[15] Gough AK, Lilley J, Eyre S, et al. Generalised bone loss in patients with early RA occurs early and relates to disease activity. Lancet 1994;344:23–7.

[16] Deodhar A, Brabyn J, Jones PW, et al. Longitudinal study of hand bone densitometry in rheumatoid arthritis. Arthritis Rheum 1995;38:1204–10.

[17] Devlin J, Lilley J, Gough A, et al. Clinical associations with DXA measurement of hand bone mass in rheumatoid arthritis. Br J Rheumatol 1996;35:1256–62.

[18] Plant MJ, Williams AL, O'Sullivan MM, et al. Relationship between time-integrated C-reactive protein levels and radiologic progression in patients with rheumatoid arthritis. Arthritis Rheum 2001;43:1473–7.

[19] Mulherin D, Fitzgerald O, Bresnihan B. Clinical improvement and radiological deterioration in rheumatoid arthritis: evidence that the pathogenesis of synovial inflammation and articular damage may differ. Br J Rheumatol 1996;35:1263–8.

[20] Conaghan PG, O'Connor P, McGonagle D, et al. Elucidation of the relationship between synovitis and bone damage: a randomized magnetic resonance imaging study of individual joints in patients with early rheumatoid arthritis. Arthritis Rheum 2003;48:64–71.

[21] Boers M, Kostense PJ, Verhoeven AC, et al, and the COBRA Trial Group. Inflammation and damage in an individual joint predict further damage in that joint in patients with early rheumatoid arthritis. Arthritis Rheum 2001;44:2242–6.

[22] Anderson JJ, Wells G, Verhoeven AC, et al. Factors predicting response to treatment in rheumatoid arthritis: the importance of disease duration. Arthritis Rheum 2000;43:22–9.

[23] Munro R, Hampson R, McEntergart A, et al. Improved functional outcome in patients with early rheumatoid arthritis treated with intramuscular gold: results of a five year prospective study. Ann Rheum Dis 1998;57:88–93.

[24] Egsmose C, Lund B, Borg G, et al. Patients with early arthritis benefit from early 2nd line therapy: 5 year follow-up of a prospective double blind placebo controlled study. J Rheumatol 1995;22:2208–13.

[25] Van der Heide A, Jacobs JWG, Bijlsma JWJ, et al. The effectiveness of early treatment with 'second-line' anti-rheumatic drugs: a randomised controlled trial. Ann Intern Med 1996; 124:699–707.

[26] Fries J, Williams CA, Morfield D, et al. Reduction in long-term disability in patients with rheumatoid arthritis by disease-modifying antirheumatic drug-based treatment strategies. Arthritis Rheum 1996;39:616–22.

[27] Abu-Shakra M, Toker R, Flusser D, et al. Clinical and radiographic outcomes of rheumatoid arthritis patients not treated with disease modifying drugs. Arthritis Rheum 1998;41:1190–5.

[28] Symmons D, Jones MA, Scott DL, et al. Long term mortality outcome in patients with rheumatoid arthritis: early presenters continue to do well. J Rheumatol 1998;25:1072–7.

[29] Green MJ, Marzo-Ortega H, McGonagle D, et al. Persistence of mild early inflammatory arthritis: the importance of disease duration, rheumatoid factor and the shared epitope. Arthritis Rheum 1999;42:2184–8.

[30] Salmon M, Emery P, Wordsworth BP, et al. Dw4 is associated with persistence but not induction of arthritis. Br J Rheumatol 1989;28(Suppl 2):79.

[31] Mottenen T, Hannonen P, Korpela M, et al. Delay in institution of therapy of remission using single-drug or combination-disease-modifying antirheumatic drug therapy in early rheumatoid arthritis. Arthritis Rheum 2002;46:894–8.

[32] Lard LR, Boers M, Verhoeven A, et al. Early and aggressive treatment of rheumatoid arthritis patients affects the association of HLA class II antigens with progression of joint damage. Arthritis Rheum 2002;46:899–905.

[33] Boers M, Verhoeven AC, Markusse HM, et al. Randomised comparison of combined step-down prednisolone, methotrexate and sulphasalazine with sulphasalazine alone in early rheumatoid arthritis. Lancet 1997;350:309–18.

[34] Landewe RB, Boers M, Verhoeven AC, et al. COBRA combination therapy in patients with early rheumatoid arthritis: long-term structural benefits of a brief intervention. Arthritis Rheum 2002;46:347–56.

[35] Quinn MA, Conaghan PG, Greenstein A, et al. Very early infliximab in addition to methotrexate in early poor prognosis rheumatoid arthritis reduces MRI synovitis and damage with sustained benefit after infliximab withdrawal: results from a double blind placebo-controlled trial. Arthritis Rheum 2005;52:27–35.

[36] St Clair EW, van der Heijde DMFM, Smolen J, et al. Combination of infliximab and methotrexate therapy for early rheumatoid arthritis: a randomised, controlled trial. Arthritis Rheum 2004;50:3432–43.

[37] Breedveld FC, Kavanaugh A, Cohen S, et al. Early treatment of rheumatoid arthritis with adalimumab plus methotrexate versus adalimumab alone or methotrexate alone: the PREMIER study. Arthritis Rheum 2004;50:4096.

[38] Bathon JM, Martin RW, Fleischmann RM, et al. A comparison of etanercept and methotrexate in patients with early rheumatoid arthritis. N Engl J Med 2000;343:1586–93.

[39] Genovese MC, Bathon JM, Martin RW, et al. Etanercept versus methotrexate in patients with early rheumatoid arthritis: two-year radiographic and clinical outcomes. Arthritis Rheum 2002; 46:1443–50.

[40] Klareskog L, van der Heijde D, de Jager JP, et al. Therapeutic effect of the combination of etanercept and methotrexate compared with each treatment alone in patients with rheumatoid arthritis: double blind randomised controlled trial. Lancet 2004;363:675–81.

[41] Klareskog L, van der Heijde D, de Jager JP, et al. Clinical outcome of a double-blind study of etanercept and methotrexate, alone and combined, in patients with active RA (TEMPO trial), year 2 results. Ann Rheum Dis 2004;63(Suppl 1):58.

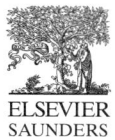

ELSEVIER
SAUNDERS

Rheum Dis Clin N Am 31 (2005) 773–796

RHEUMATIC
DISEASE CLINICS
OF NORTH AMERICA

Cumulative Index 2005

Note: Page numbers of article titles are in **boldface** type.

0889-857X/05/$ – see front matter © 2005 Elsevier Inc. All rights reserved.
doi:10.1016/S0889-857X(05)00085-2

United States Postal Service
Statement of Ownership, Management, and Circulation

1. Publication Title	2. Publication Number	3. Filing Date
Rheumatic Diseases Clinics of North America	0 8 8 9 - 8 5 7 X	9/15/05

4. Issue Frequency	5. Number of Issues Published Annually	6. Annual Subscription Price
Feb, May, Aug, Nov	4	$180.00

7. Complete Mailing Address of Known Office of Publication *(Not printer) (Street, city, county, state, and ZIP+4)*

Elsevier, Inc.
6277 Sea Harbor Drive
Orlando, FL 32887-4800

Contact Person
Gwen C. Campbell

Telephone
215-239-3685

8. Complete Mailing Address of Headquarters or General Business Office of Publisher *(Not printer)*

Elsevier, Inc., 360 Park Avenue South, New York, NY 10010-1710

9. Full Names and Complete Mailing Addresses of Publisher, Editor, and Managing Editor *(Do not leave blank)*

Publisher *(Name and complete mailing address)*

Tim Griswold, Elsevier, Inc., 1600 John F. Kennedy Blvd., Suite 1800, Philadelphia, PA 19103-2899

Editor *(Name and complete mailing address)*

Barton Dudlick, Elsevier, Inc., 1600 John F. Kennedy Blvd., Suite 1800, Philadelphia, PA 19103-2899

Managing Editor *(Name and complete mailing address)*

Heather Cullen, Elsevier, Inc., 1600 John F. Kennedy Blvd., Suite 1800, Philadelphia, PA 19103-2899

10. Owner *(Do not leave blank. If the publication is owned by a corporation, give the name and address of the corporation immediately followed by the names and addresses of all stockholders owning or holding 1 percent or more of the total amount of stock. If not owned by a corporation, give its name and address as well as those of each individual owner. If the publication is published by a nonprofit organization, give its name and address.)*

Full Name	Complete Mailing Address
Wholly owned subsidiary of	4520 East-West Highway
Reed/Elsevier, US Holdings	Bethesda, MD 20814

11. Known Bondholders, Mortgagees, and Other Security Holders Owning or Holding 1 Percent or More of Total Amount of Bonds, Mortgages, or Other Securities. If none, check box ► ☐ None

Full Name	Complete Mailing Address
N/A	

12. Tax Status *(For completion by nonprofit organizations authorized to mail at nonprofit rates) (Check one)*
The purpose, function, and nonprofit status of this organization and the exempt status for federal income tax purposes:
☐ Has Not Changed During Preceding 12 Months
☐ Has Changed During Preceding 12 Months *(Publisher must submit explanation of change with this statement)*

(See Instructions on Reverse)

PS Form 3526, October 1999

13. Publication Title	14. Issue Date for Circulation Data Below
Rheumatic Disease Clinics of North America	May 2005

15.	Extent and Nature of Circulation	Average No. Copies Each Issue During Preceding 12 Months	No. Copies of Single Issue Published Nearest to Filing Date
a.	Total Number of Copies *(Net press run)*	2975	2900
b. Paid and/or Requested Circulation	(1) Paid/Requested Outside-County Mail Subscriptions Stated on Form 3541. *(Include advertiser's proof and exchange copies)*	1396	1352
	(2) Paid In-County Subscriptions Stated on Form 3541 *(Include advertiser's proof and exchange copies)*		
	(3) Sales Through Dealers and Carriers, Street Vendors, Counter Sales, and Other Non-USPS Paid Distribution	672	699
	(4) Other Classes Mailed Through the USPS		
c.	Total Paid and/or Requested Circulation *[Sum of 15b. (1), (2), (3), and (4)]* ►	2068	2051
d. Free Distribution by Mail *(Samples, compliment-ary, and other free)*	(1) Outside-County as Stated on Form 3541	72	88
	(2) In-County as Stated on Form 3541		
	(3) Other Classes Mailed Through the USPS		
e.	Free Distribution Outside the Mail *(Carriers or other means)*		
f.	Total Free Distribution *(Sum of 15d. and 15e.)* ►	72	88
g.	Total Distribution *(Sum of 15c. and 15f.)* ►	2140	2139
h.	Copies not Distributed	835	761
i.	Total *(Sum of 15g. and h.)* ►	2975	2900
j.	Percent Paid and/or Requested Circulation *(15c. divided by 15g. times 100)*	97%	96%

16. Publication of Statement of Ownership
☐ Publication required. Will be printed in the **November 2005** issue of this publication. ☐ Publication not required

17. Signature and Title of Editor, Publisher, Business Manager, or Owner

[signature]
Joseph Panucci – Executive Director of Subscription Services

Date
9/15/05

I certify that all information furnished on this form is true and complete. I understand that anyone who furnishes false or misleading information on this form or who omits material or information requested on the form may be subject to criminal sanctions (including fines and imprisonment) and/or civil sanctions (including civil penalties).

Instructions to Publishers

1. Complete and file one copy of this form with your postmaster annually on or before October 1. Keep a copy of the completed form for your records.
2. In cases where the stockholder or security holder is a trustee, include in items 10 and 11 the name of the person or corporation for whom the trustee is acting. Also include the names and addresses of individuals who are stockholders who own or hold 1 percent or more of the total amount of bonds, mortgages, or other securities of the publishing corporation. In item 11, if none, check the box. Use blank sheets if more space is required.
3. Be sure to furnish all circulation information called for in item 15. Free circulation must be shown in items 15d, e, and f.
4. Item 15h, Copies not Distributed, must include (1) newsstand copies originally stated on Form 3541, and returned to the publisher, (2) estimated returns from news agents, and (3), copies for office use, leftovers, spoiled, and all other copies not distributed.
5. If the publication had Periodicals authorization as a general or requester publication, this Statement of Ownership, Management, and Circulation must be published; it must be printed in any issue in October or, if the publication is not published during October, the first issue printed after October.
6. In item 16, indicate the date of the issue in which this Statement of Ownership will be published.
7. Item 17 must be signed.

Failure to file or publish a statement of ownership may lead to suspension of Periodicals authorization.

PS Form 3526, October 1999 *(Reverse)*

Changing Your Address?

Make sure your subscription changes too! When you notify us of your new address, you can help make our job easier by including an exact copy of your Clinics label number with your old address (see illustration below.) This number identifies you to our computer system and will speed the processing of your address change. Please be sure this label number accompanies your old address and your corrected address—you can send an old Clinics label with your number on it or just copy it exactly and send it to the address listed below.

We appreciate your help in our attempt to give you continuous coverage. Thank you.

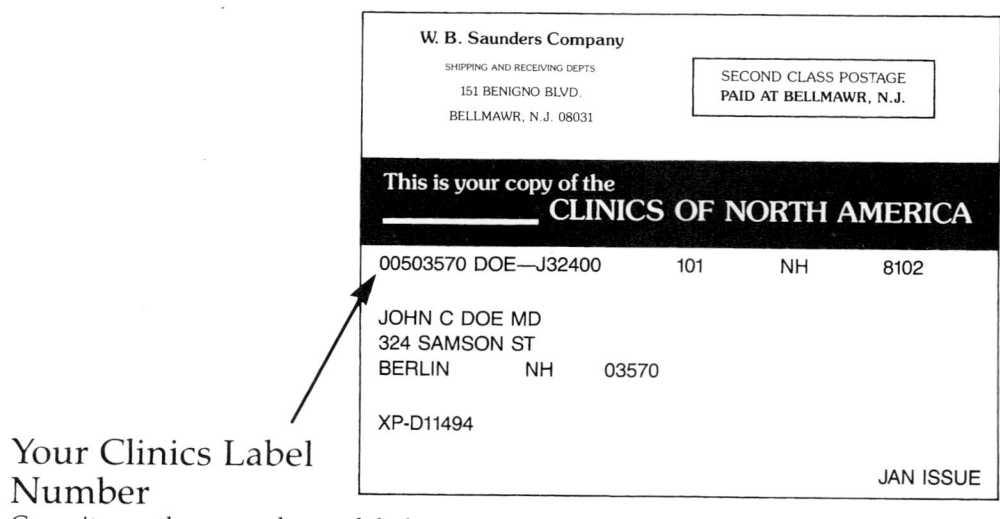

W. B. Saunders Company

SHIPPING AND RECEIVING DEPTS.
151 BENIGNO BLVD.
BELLMAWR, N.J. 08031

SECOND CLASS POSTAGE
PAID AT BELLMAWR, N.J.

This is your copy of the
_____ CLINICS OF NORTH AMERICA

00503570 DOE—J32400   101   NH   8102

JOHN C DOE MD
324 SAMSON ST
BERLIN   NH   03570

XP-D11494

JAN ISSUE

Your Clinics Label Number
Copy it exactly or send your label along with your address to:
W.B. Saunders Company, Customer Service
Orlando, FL 32887-4800
Call Toll Free 1-800-654-2452

Please allow four to six weeks for delivery of new subscriptions and for processing address changes.